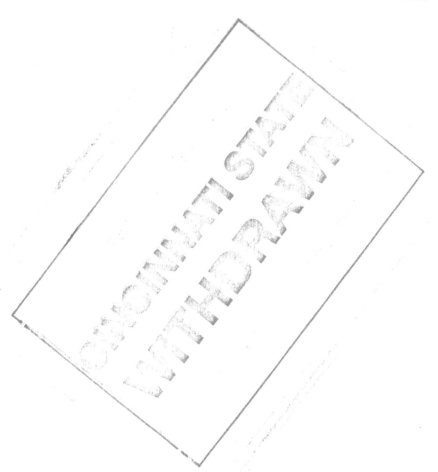

THE
HOT FLASH
COOKBOOK

THE HOT

CATHY LUCHETTI

FLASH COOK BOOK

Foreword by Risa Kagan, M.D.

Recipe Development and Consultation by Linda Hillel

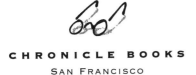

CHRONICLE BOOKS

SAN FRANCISCO

To Peter, who can take the heat

Copyright © 1997 by Cathy Luchetti.
Foreword copyright © 1997 by Risa Kagan, M.D.
All rights reserved. No part of this book may be reproduced in any form without written permission from the publisher.

Library of Congress Cataloging-in-Publication Data:
Luchetti, Cathy, 1945–
    The hot flash cookbook: delicious recipes for health and well-being
  through menopause/by Cathy Luchetti; foreword by Risa Kagan.
       p.   cm.
    Includes bibliographical references and index.
    ISBN 0–8118–1540–4 (pb)
    1. Menopause–Complications–Diet therapy–Recipes. I. Title.
RG186.L83 1997
618.1'750654–dc21

                                              97–6982
                                                 CIP

Printed in the United States of America.

Design and typesetting by Claudia Smelser
Illustrations by Leigh Wells

Distributed in Canada by Raincoast Books
8680 Cambie Street
Vancouver, British Columbia V6P 6M9

10 9 8 7 6 5 4 3 2 1

Chronicle Books
85 Second Street
San Francisco, California 94105

Web Site: www.chronbooks.com

ACKNOWLEDGMENTS

In creating this book, my warmest thanks go to Dr. Barbara Molle, who sparked the "Flash" idea and helped in its nourishing. As the idea grew, so did the enthusiasm and participation of many cheerful and intrepid friends and gourmands who sampled, cooked, and offered opinions as attendees and chefs at a near-constant round of Hot Flash dinners: Eli Leon, Steve Louie, Pat King, Georgia and Brian Moran, Don Condon, Beverly Galloway, Chris Curtis, Linda Hillel, Jon Eisenberg, Clark Finkbiner, Margaret Hungerford, Joanna Lynch, Mark Youdall, Lisa Halperin, David Austin, Eric Wogsberg, and Glenna Matthews. Special thanks to Susan Snyder and Richard Neidhardt and their children for their talented evaluations and cooking acumen; to Marian and Eric Spector for computer magic at just the right moment; to Georgia Moran and Don Lyon for inspiration, and to Lalia Mohamed of Couscous Royale, Berkeley, for a traditional Algerian recipe; to nutritionist and professor David Stone for research contributions; to Beth Hurwich for her timely recommendations as well as a stunning red "Hot Flash" apron; to Pat Cody for making available her archive of DES materials; to Leigh Roth, for research; to David Miller for support, warm friendship, and getaway inspiration; to Erin Williams and, particularly, to Linda Hillel for assiduous, creative, and careful recipe creation, testing, and advice.

Particular thanks to Dr. Susan Lark, whose informative books, including *The Menopause Self Help Book*, have been both a source of inspiration and valuable reference; to my editor Leslie Jonath; and special thanks to my agent, Anne Edelstein, whose sense of humor supported and helped put in place the Hot Flash idea.

CONTENTS

FOREWORD

In the year 1900, the average life expectancy for women was 48 years. The average life expectancy now is 82.8 years. In 1900, 45 million women were in the post-menopausal years. It has been estimated that by the year 2040, 65 million women will be over 56 and 10 million over age 85.

In 1996, the first baby boomer turned fifty years old. It is estimated that every eight seconds thereafter, another turns fifty. There will come a time in which 66 million baby boomers create a massive "senior boom."

Women are living longer and want to live the last third of their lives being healthy and active. The big question is how we want to live these years and what we can do to prevent the diseases that took the lives of our mothers and grandmothers.

The average age of menopause is fifty-one. Menopause is the culmination of a ten- to fifteen-year phase of life called the climacteric. In this phase, the production rate of estrogen and progesterone in a woman's ovaries can fluctuate. Overt symptoms such as hot flashes and irregular menstrual cycles are the hallmark of this phase. Osteoporosis and heart disease may silently be developing during this time as well.

For the past fifteen years I have had the privilege of caring for women during their reproductive and postmenopausal years. For many women, menopause is the beginning of a special time in their life. It marks the end of their periods, cramps, and PMS. They can enjoy sexual freedom, particularly freedom from pregnancy. Many women enjoy emotional and financial security because they are established in their careers and free of the responsibilities of raising children. There are women who actually describe this time of life as the "golden years." For other women, these years can be filled with debilitating emotional and physical changes. Some common questions among such women are: How do I stay healthy in this last third of life? Should I undergo hormone replacement therapy (HRT)? What can I do to prevent the common maladies of the post-menopausal years, such as heart disease, osteoporosis, cancer, and Alzheimer's disease? The answers to these questions are not easy. What is right for one individual may not be right for another. The risks versus the benefits for each individual must be carefully reviewed.

In the past, hormone replacement therapy has been prescribed for many menopausal women, because the use of the supplemental estrogen seems to solve a number of problems. Hot flashes, sleep disturbances, depression, urinary complaints, and multiple other "menopausal" symptoms are effectively reversed with HRT. Studies consistently have shown a 40 to 50 percent reduction in heart disease, the number-one cause of death for women, for patients taking HRT.

The accelerated bone loss caused by the natural decline in estrogen during menopause is also reversed by HRT. Numerous well-established studies confirm a 50 percent reduction of hip fractures if treatment begins at menopause. Some newer studies suggest that estrogen treatment begun even at age seventy or older may prevent some devastating fractures. Recent studies also suggest a decrease in colon cancer, Alzheimer's disease, and memory loss in HRT users.

With so many positive benefits, why do many women hesitate to take the supplemental estrogen? For many women the standard hormone regimens can cause undesirable side effects. There are multiple types and dosages of estrogen and progesterone. It can take six to nine months of adjustment to reach an equilibrium. For most women, the major drawback of HRT is the well-publicized potential risk of breast cancer.

Baby boomers are especially scared of breast cancer. Most menopausal women have a friend, colleague, or relative who has been affected by this most common form of cancer for women, with an incidence of one in eight women. Confusing the issue are conflicting and highly controversial studies about HRT and its risk of causing breast cancer. In 1995, two well-designed studies were published within one month of each other. One showed an increased risk of breast cancer with HRT use; the other showed no increased risk.

The short- and long-term benefits of HRT are still being studied. The National Institutes of Health has launched the Women's Health Initiative, a fifteen-year study that will, it is hoped, give us some answers. The development of the North American Menopause Society, devoted to research and education about postmenopausal women, should provide more concrete data. Unfortunately, these efforts will not provide definitive answers for several years. Our daughters and granddaughters will be the main beneficiaries of this research.

The choice of whether or not to take HRT is highly individualized. This personal decision should be reevaluated yearly with your doctor. Your lifestyle and health may change from year to year, and new data will continue to emerge.

Whatever your decision regarding HRT, a healthy diet is essential and can prove beneficial. For many years, scientists have observed that compounds in certain plant foods have structures similar to estrogen. These phytochemicals (plant-related chemicals) can block or enhance estrogen action in the body. Although they are much weaker than supplemental estrogen, they may prevent postmenopausal symptoms and diseases. Many studies are currently underway to evaluate the benefits of these food sources.

As a clinician, I have often been intrigued by the differences in menopausal symptoms among various patient populations. It is now well established that women in certain cultures with diets rich in phytochemicals, such as isoflavones (found in soybeans), have fewer menopausal symptoms. This may also explain the very low incidence of breast and prostate cancer in Asian populations. The fruits and vegetables in this diet are also rich in antioxidants, which may be helpful in protecting against heart disease and cancer.

My overall advice to my women patients is to become an informed and active participant in their health-care options, to exercise regularly, and to eat a well-balanced diet rich in foods recommended in this book. Carefully researched and brimming with useful and delicious recipes, *The Hot Flash Cookbook* is my prescription for beginning a healthy life.

—Risa Kagan, M.D.

PREFACE

For me, midlife dawned unexpected, and all too early, with the onset of the first hot flash—a startling event that suddenly defined the smaller, less visible changes that had mounted over the previous several years. The once-dependable body that had borne children, knifed down ski slopes, climbed mountains, run daily, and swum miles turned oddly unpredictable. Sighs and whispers breezed about; joints creaked, skin dried, hair turned brittle, and worst of all, my usual carefree equanimity slipped away. I was nervous about the recurring hot flashes that attacked at the least appropriate time, and that seemed sentient and devious in the manner reserved for hard drives and modems. Was there some pattern that could act as a predictor? The erratic attacks came in hot waves, breaking into a red, angry, sweating Morse code—some inner flashing of a midlife message that was incomprehensible at best, uncomfortable always, and only occurred at peak embarrassing moments.

What was happening? As a historian, I had read countless Victorian descriptions of menopause, called "the climacteric," and found them quaint and somehow touching, representing an awkward modesty and medical ignorance so profound that, in some cases, women had to point to the offending symptoms using a doll, rather than relating it to their own bodies. Daniel Turner, writing in 1714, captured the sensations of the hot flash: "Each pore looks like a little fountain, and the Sweat may be seen to stand there as clear as Rock Water, and as often as it is wiped off, to spring up . . . again."

No wonder these foremothers were thought to become "thoroughly unhinged by the change of life . . . " as well as to exhibit "low spirits and melancholy . . . and the irregularities of the passions." For the lucky ones, menopause was "a colorless, uneventful experience" during which "the ovaries, after long years of service . . . became irritated . . . [resulting in] extreme nervousness or in an outburst of actual insanity."

Droll sentiments from a bygone era? Or canny predictors of what lay ahead? Oddly enough, I felt as artless and uninformed about menopause as any Victorian matron, since nothing in my own history had prepared me for the brick-wall intransigence of midlife and its pervasive discomforts.

HRT—hormone replacement therapy—was automatically recommended. Not only would hormones give a shine to my complexion and guard against osteoporotic decline, but they offered countless benefits to the cardiovascular system. After years of living a pill-free life, I now faced a lifelong regimen of estrogen and progesterone doses, along with the fitful return of a menstrual cycle and vague fears about breast cancer. And worse, the pills induced a bloated, waxy feeling, as if I had been hormonally inflated, then dipped in butter. What were the alternatives?

As a veteran researcher, I went to the libraries, tapped into Medline, read the latest studies, talked to chemists and nutritionists, and found that the use of natural plant estrogens to boost the body's hormonal levels was, by this time, no longer experimental. "The principle that plants can produce substances with estrogenic properties was well established by 1966," wrote John Riddle (*Contraception and Abortion from the Ancient World to the Renaissance*, Harvard University Press). Phytochemical wisdom filled academic and popular journals, as well as many health and fitness magazines, offering an attractive alternative to an HRT regimen.

Yet despite the plethora of information, nutritional recommendations for menopause and, particularly, to alleviate hot flashes, seemed paltry—a cookbook was called for. Continued research, expert culinary advice, and repeated nightly bouts of sweats and hot flashes drove the idea forward.

Tentatively, I decided on a regimen of phytoestrogenic and vitamin E–rich foods, hoping that the smaller, more sedate forms of natural estrogens would provide a trigger to my own body's stored supply. I drew inspiration from Dr. Susan Lark's *The Menopause Self Help Book* and enlisted the talents of recipe consultant Linda Hillel and good friend Georgia Moran to create numerous savory dishes that were at the same time nutritionally sound and pleasing to the palate.

I started to eat dishes that were high in vitamin E and phytoestrogen, particularly fennel, yams, and tofu. Slowly, over a matter of weeks, the hot flashes seemed to recede. Tonic teas also provided soothing relief. Occasionally, there would be a flash, but like geological aftershocks, they eventually lessened. My cravings for salt and sweets also declined as I snacked on vegetables and other natural foods. A deeper feeling of health and balance prevailed, which became in turn its own reward. Why hadn't I started this years ago?

The recipes were also enjoyed by friends and family at a series of Hot Flash dinners. Even my male friends enjoyed the tasty food and the chance to discuss midlife concerns. Guests often contributed their own recipes, finding even more creative ways to feature these healthy foods. The Hot Flash dinners brought together all ages and both genders to celebrate, exchange helpful facts, and describe experiences with monopause—a forum that connected people as would any life passage in any tribe.

Thus grew the premise for this cookbook. I had learned that my physical misery could be tamed by food, that the food could be artful, elegant, and nutritious, and that the recipes could be shared with the people I loved. I had discovered the benefits of taking charge of my own midlife passage through a regimen of natural foods, and to set out to enjoy this important time of life in the best of health. I hope that *The Hot Flash Cookbook* will do the same for you.

INTRODUCTION

By the year 2000, more than 40 million women from the baby boom generation, or close to 38 percent of the population of the United States, will have reached the age of fifty. By 2015, this number will climb to 45 percent. Of these, 75 percent will experience "medium" hot flashes, and 15 percent of these hot flashes will be severely distressing, creating a huge group of women with transitional hormonal concerns. Today, approximately 14 percent of American women over the age of forty-five are taking supplemental estrogens, at no small medical expense. Given the sheer number of baby boom women, menopause is one of *the* lifestyle issues of the nineties. It is being swiftly taken up by the largest and best-educated generation of women in the country's history, who are responding to a new kind of health care: climacteric medicine.

The word *climacteric* is based on a Greek word meaning "step of a ladder." Interestingly, it was originally a medical term for a condition found in men. Eventually, the term evolved to encompass that "critical" time in a woman's life, with the final, so-called grand climacteric change falling during the sixty-third year. During the late 1800s, the word came to represent female midlife transition, with menopause cited as one part of the process. It was frequently called a "disease" in writings of the 1800s, and no amount of sympathy or assurance could convince menopausal "victims" otherwise. By 1976, as cited by anthropologist Margaret Lock, the official dictionary definition of *climacteric* was "a phase in the aging process of women marking the transition from the reproductive stage of life to the nonreproductive stage." The climacteric begins ten to fifteen years before menopause and continues for another ten years after it.

Early accounts were veiled by medical ignorance and cultural prudery and seldom described the specific occurrence of hot flashes. In fact, menopause was often cited as a breakdown of the circulatory system. In middle-class Victorian female society, which was given to the vapors, fainting, and various mysterious "female complaints," the pesky occurrence of "heat blooms" was simply one more debility to be suffered in silence.

Ignorance fostered unusual remedies, from the ancient Egyptians' search for glandular and organ therapies to restore lost vigor, to such fashionable Victorian remedies as testicular juice! Such questionable substances were injected into men to improve vigor and vesicle action, while the recommended rejuvenatives for women were juices, powders, and tablets made from animal ovaries.

In the late twentieth century, the female aging process is still considered abnormal, to be treated by regular doses of pure estrogen, the so-called youth hormone. Not only can supplemental estrogen counter hot flashes, but it restores youthful balance and prevents osteoporosis and coronary heart disease in high-risk women. Despite such claims, nearly every peak of estrogen enthusiasm has been followed by an outbreak of startling and dangerous symptoms. Introduced in the late 1940s, estrogen was a part of diethylstilbestrol (DES), the drug that was prescribed to prevent miscarriage but caused congenital abnormalities, particularly infertility. Later, estrogen returned as a contraceptive but was linked to breast cancer, blood clots, heart attacks, and liver disease. By the 1970s, estrogen was one of the country's five most frequently prescribed drugs, a wonder hormone that would keep women feminine forever. Progesterone, which mimicked the hormonal tides of the menstrual cycle, was eventually added to the prescription. But medical concerns and questions still lurked, becoming linked over time with such life-threatening diseases as endometrial cancer and gall bladder disease.

Today, women in the throes of midlife, awaiting the onset of menopause, face several unnerving possible prospects: Estrogen deprivation can induce insomnia, nervousness, depression, dizziness, fatigue, backache, loss of memory, heart palpitations, vaginal dryness, loss of libido, weight gain or loss, dry skin, blurred vision, incontinence, and hot flashes. Yet hormone replacement therapy (HRT), used to reduce some of these symptoms—and often administered in unnecessarily high doses—brings the attendant threat of endometrial cancer. According to a Nurses' Health Study, the use of estrogen by high-risk women, i.e., women with a family history of breast cancer, greatly increases their risk of breast cancer. There are also all the possible unpleasant side effects of estrogen use, including water retention and monthly bleeding.

Without HRT, however, comes the threat of estrogen-deficiency disorders, including osteoporosis, heart disease, and even Alzheimer's disease, which recent studies have linked to positive estrogenic response. Both HRT and nontreatment, then, have side effects that are often distressing and sometimes dangerous. Women already grappling with the problems of midlife are plunged into the depths of a clinical conundrum: to take HRT, or not?

There is some good news, however; recently the field of choice has broadened. Herbal, naturopathic, and culinary options are all being explored in the quest for hormonal balance. Life cycle changes, once considered to be pathological, are now viewed as normal, and can often be treated nutritionally. They are even celebrated as a step *up* the ladder of life development, rather than down.

From a vast literature, both scientific and anecdotal, comes a low-profile, nonprescription adjunct to symptom control: namely, the humble yam and a host of other plants with phytochemical activity, some bearing compounds identified as phytoestrogens. *(Phyto* is the Greek word for plants.) These and other phytoestrogenic foods, such as soybeans and flaxseeds, which are readily available at every local grocery store, can often quell the fieriest hot flash and soothe the anxious or irritable soul. Also rich in estrogen-prompting compounds are bok choy, kale, mustard greens, radishes, and blackberries, plus a host of other foods that lend a natural presence to the complex realm of hormone balancing. "It's the most exciting development in decades," says dietitian Barbara Smith, an assistant professor of food science and nutrition at Colorado State University, who believes that plant-based hormones will "usher in a golden age of health."

Phytoestrogens bear a striking resemblance to human estrogen, and exist in at least three hundred plants. Not only can these "mock" estrogens temper hot flashes and even out mood swings, but they are reported to slow the onset of osteoporosis and reduce the risk of breast cancer—and here's the best news—without all the negative side effects.

Slowly the scientific community is coming around to accepting the efficacy of natural estrogen. As long ago as 1943, Dr. Russell Marker created two kilos of the female hormone progesterone from the wild Mexican yam. Until 1970, the yam provided the only established source of diosgenin, a hormonal material used to make contraceptive pills. In the *British Medical Journal* of October 20, 1990, Australian researchers describe a photogenic (plant) experiment in which twenty-five postmenopausal women ate foods rich in plant estrogens; after six weeks, women who consumed soy flour and linseed (both estrogen-intensive) showed signs of a modest estrogen response, such as milder or reduced hot flashes and the alleviation of depression. The direct relationship between soy and estrogenic properties has been shown in many studies, including that of P. C. Kao, reported in the Chinese medical journal, *Mardi,* 1995.

Phytoestrogens are plant-based compounds designed to protect the plant from bacteria and insects. An emerging body of scientific evidence now points to the value of plant chemicals, or phytochemicals, which are neither vitamins nor minerals, but are structurally similar to estrogens. Like estrogen, they display an affinity for the hormone-binding sites of the human estrogen receptor. This mild form of estrogen found in plants is generally too weak to prevent bone loss but excels in combating hot flashes, and studies have shown that naturally occurring phytoestrogens have dramatic estrogenic effects at natural dietary levels. Herbs that contain phytoestrogens are called "adaptogenic," which means they stimulate the body's immune system to encourage self-regulation. Adaptogenic herbs with plant estrogens are used to treat hot flashes, anxiety, depression, night sweats, and insomnia.

But the question remains: Are plant estrogens enough? Plant estrogens are milder than pharmaceutical forms. Dong quai, for example, contains plant estrogens 1/400th as strong as pharmaceutical doses. Some phytoestrogens are highly effective, particularly soybean isoflavones made up of diadzein, genistein, and equol. Diets high in soy protein contain extremely high levels of isoflavones. However, these compounds are still weak estrogens, having only 1/500th to 1/1000th the biological activity of estradiol.

Yet the effects are demonstrable. In one study, women were fed 60 grams of soy protein a day for one month. Individual menstrual cycles lengthened by one to five days and cholesterol levels dropped 10 percent. Soy phytoestrogens have proven effective, with researchers agreeing that it would take 45 to 50 milligrams daily to affect a hormone cycle, with 0.5 to 2 mg. of isoflavones per gram of soy.

It is also important to remember that plant estrogens are useless without the proper accompanying diet. Choose foods wisely: fruit rather than sugar, baked or steamed foods rather than fried; less alcohol, coffee, and salt.

In addition to having high levels of phytoestrogenic activity, yams, mangoes, millet, kale, peanuts, and a dozen or so additional foods also contain large amounts of vitamin E. As sources of natural estrogen, vitamin E, and bioflavonoids—nutrients found in citrus fruits that have chemical activity similar to estrogen—these foods help to quell many distressing menopausal symptoms such as night sweats, irritability, anxiety, and irregular vaginal bleeding by replacing minute amounts of the body's depleted store of estrogen.

Whenever blood vessels constrict, a vasomotor instability occurs that is believed to be the cause of migraine headaches. Vitamin E seems to have a soothing effect on this network of nerves that control the expansion and contraction of blood vessels. Recent research has shown that vitamin E boosts energy by oxygenating cells of the body. These antioxidant properties are particularly abundant in the cruciferous vegetables: Brussels sprouts, cabbage, cauliflower, kale, turnips, and broccoli. As an antioxidant, vitamin E neutralizes free radicals, the deadly molecules that attach to the membranes of cells, preventing them from properly taking in nutrients and removing waste products. In the case of skin cells, this causes the loss of elasticity characteristic of aged skin. The body produces cholesterol to fight such damage, which triggers further oxidation, and thus more radicals.

Vitamin E also improves certain skin conditions, such as scleroderma or pigmented contact dermatitis, an often precancerous condition marked by severe itching and a red rash with thickened, cracked skin.

Just as calendar time is marked by the changing of the seasons, so our personal time, the ripening and progressing of life, is marked by the eventual waning of our reproductive abilities. Women go through this change first, while older males may maintain fertility for up to a decade or longer. The first known references to menopause date back to biblical and even prebiblical writings, but social and cultural attitudes toward "the Change" have differed greatly throughout human history.

For example, among the Quemant, an Ethiopian peasant group, menopausal women are considered privileged; they may visit normally taboo village sites, and after menopause, may even handle ritual food and beverages previously forbidden to them. As older women, they have reached an age when they are "too old to sin any longer," a notion that we in the West may find offensive, but which is greatly valued by the Quemant. Older women are esteemed as sacred by the Yanomamo of South America. They are allowed to travel freely throughout their lands and are inviolate during times of warfare. Native American women gain respect after going through menopause, since they no longer lose their "wise blood." Those tribes with a grandmother's lodge welcome older women who have passed through menopause.

In America during the 1800s, a small sect known as the Hutterites was a society dominated by older women, whose wisdom drew collective admiration and who were relieved of heavy agricultural labor at the ages of forty-five to fifty. More commonly, however, during the eighteenth and nineteenth centuries, a highly descriptive and negative menopausal literature evolved in this country in which the change of life was seen as a "catastrophe" or a "female debility" credited to any number of fictitious causes. Among the most commonly ascribed symptoms were giddiness, "moral, emotional, and intellectual aberrations," and a disturbed penchant for suicide or kleptomania, particularly if the woman was "city-bred and nervous." Even more fantastic, according to anthropologist Margaret Lock, was the nineteenth-century belief that women's skulls were "narrow, childlike, and delicate," unlike the sturdy craniums of superior males. With such inherent design flaws, was it any wonder that, for such aging yet childlike creatures, biology was, indeed, destiny?

Phytoestrogens maintain their efficacy at temperatures of 350°, 430°, 490°, and 540°F. On the other hand, vitamin E is destroyed by overheating and is easily "washed" away. To capture both flavor and nutrients, E-bearing vegetables should be lightly steamed.

One thing is clear: There is a need for a broader understanding of the impact of menopause on the health and well-being of women. Because nutrition obviously plays a major part in women's health, further study of women's nutritional needs is essential.

In the "treatment" of menopausal symptoms, nutrition should be balanced with good sense. Diets should emphasize more legumes, grains, soy products, and vegetables, with sugars and salts decreased or eliminated. In "fifty-something" recipes, calcium- and vitamin E-rich foods should predominate. The pleasure of obtaining vitamins, minerals, and micronutrients from foods rather than pills, potions, acids, and other supplements is obvious. Good nutrition improves general health and well-being, which in turn influences quality of life. After all, people eat food first, not nutrients.

We consume our foods with gusto, savor the flavors, and enjoy the communion of friends and family gathered around a laden table. The idea that practical physiological changes and improvements also are effected by these foods is, if nothing else, a bonus. Food as medicine has long existed in the tribal realm, and, in recent years, in the domain of the naturopathic practitioner. Many of the touted effects of vitamin E and phytoestrogen-bearing foods are still being evaluated by Western medicine. The National Institutes of Health, the Kaiser Permanente health maintenance organization, and the Menopause Institute have launched studies that are as yet incomplete. Although an abundance of literature exists, barriers still loom between traditional and alternative medical approaches. Although many of us envision a merging of the two, the process is slow, with only a few North American medical schools incorporating alternative studies into their regular school curricula.

For now, the use of vitamin E and phytoestrogens resides in the realm of recommendation, anecdotal evidence, and enthusiastic personal testimony rather than prescription. As demand grows for sympathetic and natural treatment for a

Introduction

generation of women turning fifty, increased scientific validation will support what so many women are already experiencing: a hot-flash-free change of life, enjoyed in the company of friends and family around the dinner table.

The purpose of this cookbook is to channel dietary preoccupations back to the simple pleasures of well-prepared, easily available foods that are nutritionally sound yet also replete with the additional bonus of natural estrogenic properties.

Pharmacological foods, however, can be misused without professional guidance. In the condition identified by one scientific study as "ginseng abuse syndrome," for example, high blood pressure can result from mixing caffeine with ginseng. *The Hot Flash Cookbook* takes the worry and guesswork out of cooking and emphasizes familiar, locally available foods to be eaten with simple pleasure and without thought to dosages and degrees. With these recipes women can feel assured in the knowledge that subtle health enhancements are continually taking place.

WHAT IS MENOPAUSE?

Clouded in myth yet grounded in the reality of millions of women's experience, menopause is often defined more easily by what it is not, rather than what it is. Because the condition coincides with aging, symptoms are often confused one for the other, leaving puzzling gaps in our current practice and understanding of so-called climacteric medicine. For example, many of the symptoms associated with menopause mimic those of adrenal gland stress disorders. Interestingly, once the ovaries have ceased to function, the adrenal glands take over by producing small amounts of estrogen, and can continue in this effort for years. Yet, if the adrenals have been nutritionally depleted or unduly stressed, they are unable to function in their new capacity, creating symptoms of adrenal stress similar to those of menopause, such as irritability, fatigue, mood swings, nervous disorders, and depression.

The myths surrounding menopause are legion: that the intensity and duration of PMS earlier in life predicts a difficult menopause; that menopause itself triggers such intense mood swings that concentration is lost and self-control goes completely haywire. Stories of nervousness, sleep loss, and stress abound, yet each woman eventually finds her own level of tolerance for her symptoms, depending on her health and various hereditary factors. Some of the biggest myths surrounding menopause are the ones that relate to sexual dysfunction, including frigidity, libido loss, or inability to have sex. For some there may be a waning of the libido and vaginal dryness, but not for all. And there are treatments for both conditions, both pharmaceutical and nutritional.

Can cultural expectations influence symptoms? The question calls on anthropology as well as clinical and research medicine for answers, which are often buried in a welter of disagreement over the methods of comparing characteristics of the populations studied. Rather than differences of weight, height, and socioeconomic class, perhaps the answer lies in the fact that estrogenic plants account for 50 percent of the calories eaten in various global locales, particularly Asia, where far fewer hot flash complaints are documented.

Is menopause a biological or social phenomenon, a natural process or a disease? Interestingly, a study of 483 women in India contends that hot flashes are culturally induced since women without symptoms acquired them when they changed locations and mingled with other symptomatic women. Not all the women in the study group spoke English, and the data did not adequately reflect the outcome; however, it certainly raises the broader question: Are the menopausal symptoms reported by Westerners absent in other cultures, or are they simply perceived differently, or are they attributed to aging, rather than menopause?

Research reveals that Mexican women from the Yucatán Peninsula, who often have from twelve to seventeen pregnancies and up to fourteen live births, seldom have reported hot flashes, or any other common menopausal complaints. In Africa, hot flashes are often confused with malaria, while in Japan, where self-control and balance are considered integral to health, few women reported hot flashes in a menopausal study, although some did complain of stiff shoulders and headaches. The lack of hot flashes may be due to the ingestion of gamma oryzanol, a naturally occurring component of rice bran oil that reduces hot flashes dramatically. In fact, according to nutritionist Ann Louise Gittleman, as little as 300 milligrams of gamma oryzanol per day creates an 85 percent reduction in hot flashes. In Mexico, a daily diet of beans and corn tortillas provides a superb source of both calcium and magnesium, which contribute to healthy bones and fewer menopausal complaints.

In one of the most interesting studies, urban Westernized Javanese women were compared to migrant and rural women; hot flashes occurred more frequently in the more Western-acculturated group in the urban area and less frequently in the women living in the rural area, but when rural women migrated to the cities, hot flash incidents increased.

The onset of menopause has some possible predictors. Early menstruation as a young girl can predict a later onset of menopause, perhaps due to better ovarian function, whereas women with shorter monthly cycles may reach menopause before the average age of fifty-one. Oddly enough, from a nutritional standpoint, menopause seems easier for overweight women, although the deleterious effects of excess weight on an individual's health are far greater than the minor hormonal advantages. The body's own supply of fatty tissues continues to create and supply estrogen long after the ovaries have ceased to function. These "worker" cells busily convert other sex hormones from the ovaries and/or adrenal glands into estrogen. Such self-conversion often means fewer and less intense hot flashes as well as prolonged vaginal moisture.

Making menopause more comfortable becomes a key health decision for midlife women. As a female rite of passage, it offers a pause in life's regimen, which can be seen as a constructive, midlife hiatus: a time to take stock of weight, general physical health, bone density, cholesterol levels, uterine health, mental agility, emotional outlook, sexual drive and performance, and, underlying everything, diet. What should change? What can remain the same? Studies show that it is often premenopausal women who worry more about the event—or nonevent—than women who have actually sailed through the menopausal process.

Medically, menopause calls for an early baseline checkup to establish a norm against which future functions are measured. Blood tests, mammograms, bone-density tests, and cardiovascular fitness tests should be done. Physical changes are gradual, taking a period of years, often beginning with the first flush of a hot flash or with irregular periods. For every woman, the net health effect of the midlife passage is marked by a gradual decline in estrogen, which affects different women in different ways. Some develop PMS-type symptoms, ranging from food cravings to mood swings to bloating, while others toss and turn with night sweats or hot flashes, or experience vaginal dryness. Others have no symptoms at all, calmly shifting from pre- to postmenopause without any stress or bother. Menopause specialist Wulf Utian, M.D., Ph.D., estimates that half of all menopausal women fail to recognize menopausal symptoms, or don't have them at all. As the metabolism shifts and changes, exercise and diet become increasingly more important. Not only are bones releasing calcium at an unprecedented rate, but muscles are relaxing and losing tone, while weight can inch upward, gaining rapid momentum with every sweet indulgence, each delicious, fatty food.

Unfortunately, the natural process of aging prompts gradual loss of muscle mass and strength and an upsurge in body fat, particularly around the abdomen. Belly fat is a recognized precursor to heart disease in both men and women and is a significant postmenopausal concern. Many studies have shown that weight gain is a prime complaint, whether women are on HRT or not. A sluggish lifestyle and a slower metabolism often proceed unless checked.

What to eat? Mindfulness and moderation are more useful than food fads or obsessions, and are keyed to a woman's individual style, history, needs, tastes, and interests. Generally, the ideal regimen for the midlife woman is a low-fat, high-fiber diet scant in sugar and alcohol and free of tobacco.

Even at midlife, variety rather than obsession yields good health. Each food provides a key nutrient that builds on, or is supported by, the presence of other vitamins and minerals. Varying fruits, vegetables, meats, and grains will provide the best balance. Part of the midlife quest is to customize a biochemical "profile" that works, and to develop an appropriate and, above all, *realistic* regimen. After all, what good are lifestyle changes that no one can live with comfortably. Depending on a woman's hormonal profile, menopausal symptoms will differ radically, and the approaches that a woman may choose are individual and may change over time. Some women will opt for the higher dosage of HRT, without suffering the side effects. Others will endorse only a natural regimen, gleaning the estrogen and vitamins needed from food sources rather than pills. Some women will try a combination of both. Interestingly, many physicians report that no matter how many pills are prescribed, inevitably, women end up making their own decisions. A very large number will take the pills for a period of time, then reduce their dosage or stop completely, while others continue dosing religiously.

Exercise is essential: at least twenty minutes of aerobic exercise three times a week is indispensable for cardiovascular health. A daily regimen of an hour or more might demand more food, yet, quixotically, excess aerobic activity can *deplete* estrogen sources, revealing yet again that moderation is often the best medicine in the midlife years.

ESTROGEN

Estrogen is a hormone produced naturally in a woman's body. It is not the only hormone women produce: testosterone, progesterone (a substance produced by the ovaries), DHEA (a weak androgen produced by the adrenal gland), and a number of other natural stimulants are all part of a woman's chemical makeup.

Estrogen is the force behind a woman's sexual activity and drive from her earliest teenage years until menopause and beyond. Estrogen is a name given to a class of hormones produced by the ovaries, the three most important being estrone, estradiol, and estriol. These hormones produce an estruslike action, or sexual "heat." Peaking estrogen levels provoke the highest sexual response in young women, coinciding with their highest levels of fertility. During ovulation, estrogen levels rise and fall in exact opposition to progesterone production. If an egg is not fertilized, both estrogen and progesterone fade away, to come surging back during the next menstrual period. In earlier generations and civilizations, the waning of estrogen levels at menopause signaled the end of a woman's productive life. Today, menopause is a midlife marker for women who can happily expect to live full and healthy lives well into their postmenopausal years. During menopause, estrogen levels drop dramatically, prompting the great debate between those who believe in natural aging and those who see prolonged estrogen use as a lifeline to youth. The third alternative of dietary therapy treads gently on both sides.

Linking behavior to hormones is a touchy area, recalling past complaints about women's fitness for any number of occupations, professions, and even recreational activities. The claims of increased sexuality, restored vigor, and youthful luster due to increased estrogen levels are dramatic and seductive. Tests have shown that estrogen surges can induce higher levels of melatonin, which induces deep, restful sleep. Estrogen also improves manual dexterity and perceptual and verbal skills. According to Doreen Kimura, a behavioral endocrinologist at the University of Western Ontario, many distinctly female cognitive skills are linked to estrogen levels, and the addition of estrogen to a depleted system may slow the rate of cognitive decline. The slow diminishment of hormonal levels, cognitive thinking, and sexual vigor can be reversed, according to the latest research. Estrogen has also been shown in medical studies to restore moisture to dry skin and luster and shine to brittle hair.

Estrogen also serves as a cardiovascular sentry, guarding against heart attacks by raising levels of "good" HDL, or high-density lipoprotein, in the blood, and lowering the amount of "bad" LDL, or low-density lipoprotein. Because estrogen levels fall during menopause, the risk of heart disease rises steadily. Heart disease is the gravest health threat to American women, killing approximately 250,000 annually from heart attacks, and another 90,000 from strokes.

Claims that long-term estrogen therapy may reduce the incidence of coronary heart disease have been recently substantiated by a study by the National Institutes of Health. Estrogen was shown to reduce a variety of risk factors, including the substantial increase in levels of HDL cholesterol, lowering the risk of heart disease up to 25 percent.

Advanced studies in natural healing all point to the benefits of the synthesis of vitamins, minerals, hormones, and compounds within the body, rather than isolated applications. Nutritionally, foods far outstrip the efficacy of pills and tonics, particularly when it comes to heart disease in women. The risk of coronary heart disease, identified recently as the number-one killer of women, can be lowered significantly by replacing estrogen in the menopausally depleted body, by strict adherence to a low-fat diet, by implementing an appropriate exercise program, and by not smoking. In countries where soy is served at every meal, rates of heart disease and many forms of cancer are unusually low. In Shanghai, China, for example, the average cholesterol level hovers around 165. In the United States, the average tops 200.

None of this low-fat information is new; for the past forty years, each decade has yielded a host of dieting advice, aimed primarily at men. Yet the number of U.S. deaths from cardiovascular disease has risen since 1993, a change attributable to the aging of the large baby boom population. As "baby boomer" women approach menopause, they must become aware of a new vulnerability: a Nurses' Health Study of 32,000 postmenopausal women showed that women taking estrogen had a 70 percent to 50 percent lowered risk of heart attack over women not taking estrogen. Thus, the vitamin E-rich and estrogenic foods recommended in the following chapters can go an additional step toward heart health.

Estrogen is one of the hormones that helps to regulate fluid balance, and fluctuations of estrogen cause changes in the body's sodium level. The result is water retention in the cells, or excess water and accompanying breast tenderness, and anxiety. When estrogen fails to stimulate receptors in the urogenital system, stress incontinence may result. Low estrogen levels can also cause dryness of skin, hair, and mucous membranes as well as adversely affecting the central nervous system, resulting in sleep disorders.

Estrogen helps the bones hold calcium and other minerals. Most women lose bone mass after menopause, particularly in the first five to ten years, and particularly if they are in the high-risk categories of being thin and small-boned, or smokers, or daughters of women who had osteoporosis. A "hot flash" diet that is rich in vitamin E also supplies, through nutritious green leafy vegetables, bountiful amounts of calcium to help stabilize its constant leaching from the bones. Calcium seeps away through the urine and escapes through the skin, and is lost through excessive caffeine use, inactivity, and smoking, as well as through the deleterious effects of certain prescription and over-the-counter drugs and various chronic diseases. By midlife, the absorption of calcium into the body is slowed, causing acceleration of bone loss. Early dietary and exercise habits create dense, healthy bones, which are less prone to osteoporosis and will retain enough bone solidity and calcium to make midlife maintenance easier.

Fragile, demineralized bones presage future trouble, as well as the need for more calcium. Recent studies reveal that milk may actually help deplete calcium stores in the body. Regular milk, although rich in vitamin E, is also high in fat and is not considered a balanced food. Milk is low in fiber and has few complex carbohydrates, and whole milk can create a fat buildup in the artery walls. Large protein intake in childhood causes overly rapid bone development, thus a weakened, porous skeletal structure. However, nonfat milk has 380 milligrams of calcium and is an important dietary supplement.

What Is Menopause?

Regular exercise, particularly that which involves weight-bearing activities, and a low-protein, low-fat diet with fewer dairy products, less coffee, carbonated drinks, alcohol, salt, and sugar, and more dark green leafy vegetables, nuts, seeds, tofu, and sea vegetables such as hijiki or wakame, help to maintain bone density and inhibit the steady demineralization of the bones. Even soy sauce comes with a caution: One tablespoon of regular soy sauce equals slightly more than 1,000 milligrams of sodium. Since the recommended daily intake of sodium is, according to nutritionist Ann Louise Gittleman, only 2,000, use low-sodium soy sauce.

While calcium in the diet appears to influence whether or not a woman is at risk for bone loss, magnesium is also critical. Without magnesium, calcium fails to strengthen bones and instead becomes lodged in the joints as calcium deposits and bone spurs, causing in some cases severe, even crippling pain.

Estrogen levels at midlife seem to affect bone loss. Sufficient estrogen in the system, whether from plant sources, natural hormonal processes, or replacement therapy, facilitates calcium absorption from the digestive process as well as maintains a higher level of estrogen in the blood. The longer estrogen blankets the system, the better the protective effect on bones. However, since phytoestrogens are very weak estrogens as compared to pharmaceutical sources, they are not always entirely effective in preventing bone loss.

A Swedish study concluded that hormone therapy produced a 60 percent reduction in hip fractures. Clearly this is one of estrogen's advantages in the ongoing race between risk and benefit. But the larger question remains: to use HRT or natural dietary estrogen?

Hormone replacement therapy, or HRT, is a combination of estrogen and progesterone given in pill or patch form to stop or reduce menopausal symptoms. The most common replacement therapy is Premarin, which is made from the collected urine of pregnant mares.

There is no doubt that drugs can effectively mask menopausal symptoms, as well as flush water into the cells, which plumps up the skin, making wrinkles less obvious. HRT therapy alleviates hot flashes and lubricates the vaginal lining, improving midlife sex. A very recent study from Johns Hopkins School of

Medicine has intrigued the medical world: the evidence suggests that post-menopausal women who take estrogen (in the form of replacement drugs) run about half the risk of Alzheimer's disease as those who do not. Estrogen seems to have a protective effect against the disease, although the evidence was gained from hormone replacement therapy, rather than the ingestion of phytoestrogens.

Any woman who takes estrogen without a balancing dose of progesterone greatly increases the risk of cancer, although progesterone is nearly always given. Some synthetic progesterones cause undesirable side effects, including PMS-like symptoms such as bloating or depression. The main objection to HRT pills is the possible risk of breast cancer, thus the preference for dietary estrogen substitutes rather than synthetic.

Despite the claims of more youthful skin tone and improved memory, a survey taken in 1987 showed that up to 30 percent of women given an estrogen prescription never filled it, and of those who did, one fifth stopped the hormone after nine months, claiming miserable side effects such as water retention, mood swings, weight gain, breast tenderness, depression, and breakthrough bleeding.

In the past, HRT was routinely prescribed for menopausal women. Now individual patient profiles must be drawn, and a careful weighing of risks and benefits takes place. Ultimately, a woman must decide for herself whether hormone replacement therapy is right for her. Research continues, as does the controversy.

Although contradictory assertions are common and data sets often noncompatible, enough doubt clouds the discourse to have prompted a ten-year $500 million epidemiological study by the National Institutes of Health, involving over 140,000 women, which will attempt to explain the relationship between HRT and chronic disease.

NATURAL ESTROGENS

So, why natural estrogens? Although the amount of estrogen ingested in a prepared food such as yam soup is considerably less than that found in prescription hormones (approximately 1/50,000 the strength of commercial estrogen), even the weaker estrogenic activity has been shown to effectively combat hot flashes.

In a society in which women have ovulated and produced estrogen for many more years than their forebears because of increased lifespan, and where menopause is considered a medical condition for which estrogen is the treatment, the question arises: How much estrogen is too much? Women concerned about the intrusion of science into the natural process and who prefer limited doses of natural estrogen rather than intense hormonal flooding may prefer food therapy. Interestingly, studies have shown that the natural dietary phytoestrogen coumestrol induced extraordinary uterine growth in rats. Thus the idea that potent phytoestrogens must be considered when calculating the total estrogenic load to which humans are exposed during a normal life. With estrogens filtering in from the plant world, artificially boosting that input with additional pharmaceutical estrogen may be extreme for some women.

In fact, studies have shown that some phytoestrogens are cumulative and have dramatic estrogenic effects at normal dietary levels. Some plant estrogens, such as the phytoestrogens found in clover, alfalfa, and soybeans, are potent enough to cause reproductive toxicity in some small animals.

On the other hand, researchers have found that many hormone-dependent cancers are possibly caused by specific components of the Western diet. A semi-vegetarian diet may alter hormone production, while some hormonelike phytoestrogens found in soybean products, whole-grain cereals, seeds, and probably berries and nuts seem to play a somewhat cancer-protective role. The phytocompounds in the plants are converted to hormonelike compounds by intestinal bacteria.

Still in the very earliest stages of research is the field of xenoestrogens. These are produced outside the body but mimic the effect of estrogen on the body's cells. Such free-floating compounds are ubiquitous, often "floating" in the microscopic petrochemical pollution of the air, water, and soil. When they come into contact with hormone receptor sites in the body they may cause the body to react as if flooded with extra hormones, triggering rapid cell growth that could ultimately lead to diseases such as breast cancer and arthritis. Xenoestrogenic research remains in the speculative stage, as do parallel studies, now underway, on how to block renegade xenoestrogens.

Startling preliminary findings show that specific plant estrogens are highly effective in blocking the estrogens that cause tumor growth. These phytoestrogens are found in such commonly consumed products as oregano, goldenseal, pennyroyal, licorice, soy milk, thyme, yucca, and the plant with the strongest estrogenic activity of all, bloodroot. (Pennyroyal, goldenseal, licorice, and bloodroot are consumed as teas.)

Although much more research is needed, what *is* clear is that the system that loses estrogen is at risk of eventually developing conditions that range from the inconvenient and uncomfortable to the dangerous and even life-threatening. In addition, estrogen may affect the production of endorphins in the brain, which contributes to feelings of calm and well-being. Definite links exist between emotional states and hormonal levels during menopause. Select research projects are presently studying these links.

WHAT ARE HOT FLASHES?

Several theories exist. One is that vasomotor instability causes erratic behavior of the nerve centers and the body's blood flow, resulting in a flooding, prickling sensation. Another theory suggests that the decreased flow of estrogen and progesterone triggers an increased flow of FSH, or follicle-stimulating hormone. Pumped by the pituitary gland in an attempt to restimulate the ovaries, FSH upsets the body's glandular balance, causing a surge of heat and nervousness. Between 75 percent and 85 percent of menopausal women experience some variety of hot flash, from severe, deep, burning ones, lasting several minutes, to slight feelings of uncomfortable warmth. The most bothersome complaint for women who experience this hemodynamic change is often profuse sweating, which is localized primarily in the upper body. Flashes can occur spontaneously, or may be triggered by stress, external heat, or confining space. Many women claim that hot flashes are slightly more frequent, intense, and disturbing during the summer.

Also, body types and hot flash severity or frequency can correlate, according to two anthropologists at San Diego State University who have determined, in a nonclinical sample survey, that women with greater lower-body fat, as opposed to upper-body fat, or who had experienced menarche at a later age, tended toward more pronounced hot flashes. These so-called "flushers" also are found to have a higher level of forearm blood flow than non-flushers. Vegetarians, women who exercise vigorously, and women who are 10 percent or more over their ideal body weight are less likely to have hot flashes. Interestingly, a Swedish team has verified the benefits of acupuncture in relieving hot flashes and sweating episodes, with effects lasting up to three months.

Alternative medicine, particularly traditional Chinese medicine, identifies any bodily distress, including menopausal symptoms, as an indication of bodily imbalance. In this spirit, preliminary research in the Netherlands and Sweden revealed that severe hot flashes may be an early warning of bone loss. Of 126 women studied, 64 percent had hot flashes for one to five years, 26 percent six to ten years, and 10 percent for more than eleven years. For most women the time period for experiencing hot flashes lasts about two years, although some women in their seventies and eighties have reported hot flashes. As for frequency, ten flashes per twenty-four hours seems typical. Without treatment, hot flashes usually persist for the first several years of menopause and could last as long as five years. Interestingly, women who take estrogen therapy generally have hot flashes for a longer period of time than women who do not take estrogen, or who take natural herbal substitutes.

VITAMIN E

The so-called anti-aging vitamin is rich in antioxidants. These substances remove the "free radicals" that destroy the connective tissues beneath the skin and increase internal antioxidation. Without adequate vitamin E, cellular wastes in the blood merge with oxygen to form toxic degenerative compounds such as hydrogen peroxide. Midlife tissues are particularly subject to oxidation, which actually means decay. The more "spoilage," or oxidation, our cells support, the faster the aging process occurs. The accumulation of free radicals in brain tissue has been linked to age-related memory loss, an unfortunate sign of early aging.

The antioxidant properties of vitamin E help keep the cells from premature decay, which explains its reputed "sunscreen" ability to protect the skin from the ravages of UV exposure. Although the vitamin tested was in capsule form applied topically, not in its food form, the vitamin's proven ability to reduce the redness and tenderness of sunburn is a strong argument for its inclusion in the daily diet. A Swedish study showed improved arterial flow in a group taking vitamin E, which led to greater endurance in activities such as walking.

Vitamin E also acts as an estrogen source, turning agitated "hot flashers" into "past flashers" through a complicated series of interactions. Studies indicate that a daily dose of vitamin E over a month or more will gradually alleviate hot flashes, the muscular distress of leg cramps, and even vaginal dryness in at least *half* to *two thirds* of women surveyed. Several studies have shown vitamin E to alleviate some symptoms of PMS by affecting the production of prostaglandins, hormonelike substances in the body that regulate a myriad of processes, including reproduction, muscle contraction, and blood pressure levels.

Unlike other vitamins, E is not naturally produced in the human body, and is a generic term for several fat-soluble compounds called tocopherols and tocotrienols. Plant sources of E are preferable to animal sources because of lower fat. An active component in broccoli, asparagus, cabbage, whole grains, wheat germ, safflower oil, wheat germ oil, walnuts, filberts, peanuts, and almonds, vitamin E is also present in wakame, a sea vegetable. Soybean oil and corn oil also brim with the prized vitamin, as do mangoes, millet, and lamb, although few foods will provide the equivalent of vitamin E pills. The richest and most surprising sources of vitamin E are carrot leaves, the outer leaves of cabbage, and the outer leaves of broccoli.

Vitamin E functions best if vitamin C is also present, which is easily provided by many sources, including citrus and tomato juices.

A tangential result of vitamin E in the body, although not as unilateral as others, is its essential role in increasing iodine absorption in the body, which contributes to a healthy thyroid.

Is there such a thing as too much vitamin E? A daily capsule dose of 1,000 or more international units is purported to prevent heart disease; the larger the body size, the greater the need. A new study shows that taking a strong dose of vitamin E—about ten times the recommended daily allowance of 30 IUs—reduced plaque buildup in patients "equivalent to about fourteen years of aging," according to nutritionist Lisa Nicholson of the Southern California School of Medicine. It is important to note that even participants who did not take supplements, but who ate foods naturally rich in vitamin E, showed reductions in artery narrowing. Some people are sensitive to vitamin E—an excellent reason to take E in moderate amounts through food sources, rather than direct pill doses. **Note:** Vitamin E dissipates with freezing and overcooking.

> ### CAUTION
>
> *Vitamin E supplements should not be taken by women with a history of high blood pressure, diabetes, or rheumatic heart disease. In addition, vitamin E taken as a supplement is fat-soluble and, if taken to excess, can build up in the body, causing problems. Also, vitamin E should be taken at the end of a meal that contains fats, since it is absorbed into the intestinal tract only through fats. It should not be taken with iron supplements.*

The following common foods are grouped by the amounts of vitamin E they contain. All oils are in measurements of 1 tablespoon; vegetables are cooked in half-cup measurements.

50 IUs or more:	20 IUs or more:	10 IUs or more:	5 IUs or more:
Wheat germ oil	Corn oil	Almonds (¼ cup)	Almond oil
	Soybean oil	Filberts	Macadamia nuts
		Hazelnuts	Palm oil
		Canola oil	Peanuts
		Cottonseed oil	Soybeans
		Skim milk (8 oz.)	(½ cup, cooked)
		Sunflower oil	Sweet potato,
		Sunflower seeds	medium

50 IUs or more:	20 IUs or more:	10 IUs or more:	5 IUs or more:
		Wheat germ	Tofu (½ cup)
		Whole milk (8 oz.)	

Below 5 IUs:

Acorn squash	Spinach	Peanut butter	Cottage cheese
Asparagus	Swiss chard	(2 tbs)	Oil and vinegar
Avocado	Turnip greens	Pine nuts	dressing
Butternut squash	Apricots	Walnuts	Bass
Dandelion greens	Blueberries	Chocolate	Bluefish
Green peas	Mango	(1 oz.)	Cod
Kale	Olives, black	Bagel	Mackerel
Lima beans	Peach	Brown rice	Oysters (1 cup, raw)
Mustard greens	Prunes, dried (10)	Wild rice	Perch
Pumpkin	Cashews	Garbanzo beans	Salmon
(canned, ½ cup)	Pecans	Navy beans	Sole

MALEPAUSE

Although this cookbook caters to the midlife symptoms of women, some notice should be taken of the male equivalent, since, as quoted in *The New York Times* of October 25, 1994, "Estrogen is as important to a man's bone strength and skeletal structure as it is to a woman's." Although having nothing to do with menstruation, the midlife period of time for men (popularly called either andropause or viropause) can be as debilitating as menopause is for women, as shown by the results of a congress on the subject held in Stockholm in 1993. More than 20 percent of men over the age of fifty suffered from increased nervousness, constipation, impaired memory, reduced potency, and interestingly, excessive perspiration.

Lower hormone levels were cited as a cause for impotence, due to a weak supply of the male hormone androgen. The situation can be reversed by testosterone replacement therapy. It has been found that a testosterone booster can also increase bone density. While far more common in women, osteoporosis afflicts men as well. Male HRT also increases "good" HDL cholesterol, providing heart protection from disease as well as increased sexual potency, mental alertness, and grip strength. Contrary to popular belief, men do produce estrogen, converting it from the male hormone androgen. For men, too much estrogen causes breast growth, headaches, weight gain, and mood swings, while too little hinders the proper mineralization and growth of bones during adolescence. The role of estrogen in male skeletal structure and bone development has recently been reevaluated. Produced in the adrenal glands and testes, estrogen is "sealed" in the body through the sensitive action of estrogen sensors in the cells, and is critical to bone metabolism—growth and adequate mineralization particularly. Another widely accepted theory is that estrogen is an essential signal for shaping the male brain and the formation of sexual identity. Estrogen use in maturity possibly functions to increase insulin sensitivity and decrease the risk of cardiovascular disease.

Although male sex hormones do not decline at the same rate as women's during menopause, by their late seventies and early eighties, men have only half to a third of their youthful testosterone levels. The male hormonal profile can be enhanced in a number of ways: through stimulation of the adrenal gland, the hypothalamus, the sex glands, or the liver. Although the field of anti-aging through hormones is still in the fledgling stages, systemic similarities between men and women suggest that the same phytochemicals—phytoestrogens—and the daily use of vitamin E, either from vitamin supplements or through food sources, can be useful to men as well.

Vitamin E is a fat-soluble vitamin that protects the body from the oxidizing effects of "bad," or LDL, cholesterol breakdown—the chief cause of heart attacks. The growing literature concerning vitamin E in the prevention of heart disease stems from the Cambridge Antioxidant Study, which established that vitamin E supplements reduced the risk of heart attack by 77 percent. The controlled study included both men and women, and in both genders it was equally effective.

Some conditions are typically thought of as "women's diseases," yet they do affect a segment of the male population. As stated earlier, osteoporosis affects about 5 million men in this country, although male bone mass is considerably more dense than that of women, and bone loss begins later and develops more slowly. Many of the *Hot Flash* recipes that are rich in calcium can contribute to sustained bone density.

Surprisingly, men make up nearly fifteen hundred of the annual 183,400 new cases of breast cancer. Often, this is a result of hyperestrogenism, a disorder resulting in the abnormal flooding of estrogen in the male system. Prostate cancer, one of the most common threats to midlife men, is being linked to abnormal hormonal reactions. Yet recent studies have shown that the phytochemicals, specifically the phytomins that are found in tomatoes, have strong antioxidant and disease-preventing properties. The more tomato sauce, the less chance of prostate cancer, was the recent advice of Harvard researchers.

A major new focus of research for men centers on an important hormone, produced by the pituitary gland, called growth hormone. Whether production of this hormone can be stimulated by phytoestrogens or vitamin E-rich foods is yet to be determined. Another focus of male hormone research centers on the effort to combat the effect of declining hormones in older men. Testosterone replacement therapy, now under consideration, may prove to prevent, alleviate, or postpone chronic and debilitating illness. Such anti-aging techniques may also prove to reverse the degenerative changes in bone, muscles, nerves, and cartilage that result from hormone loss.

Gender differences fade away in the face of good nutrition, and men who are ordinarily free of the effects of hormonal depletion, namely hot flashes, can still benefit from the advantages of phytoactive and vitamin E-enriched foods. Improved skin tone and bone mass, thinner blood, and more protection from heart disease are only a few health byproducts of such a regimen for men.

HOT FLASH FOODS

Rich in phytoestrogens and vitamin E and other healthful elements, the following foods form the basis of the hot flash diet. Although some of the herbs may only be found in health food stores, most of these ingredients are available in local supermarkets.

Fish

Fish from northern waters are extremely rich in omega-3 oil, a polyunsaturated oil that is particularly useful to cardiovascular health. Omega-3 purportedly lowers the "harmful" LDL cholesterol, elevates the "good" HDL, and contributes to brain growth and development. What's its importance to menopausal women? Omega-3 oil helps to boost the immune system, and fish such as mackerel, which is high in this type of fat, also contain healthy portions of magnesium, known to relieve menopausal hot flashes as well as fatigue and depression. In research studies, when consumed in the form of flaxseed oil and fish oil, omega-3 fats reduced or eliminated a number of troublesome menopausal ailments such as vaginal dryness and depression. In addition, the oils promoted good circulation and thinner blood, and lowered the risk of heart attacks, a still controversial claim that ongoing research should soon clarify.

Fatty fish oils are found in tandem with vitamin E, which is proven to relieve the discomfort of hot flashes. The fish containing the most vitamin E are mackerel, bluefish, tuna, salmon, butterfish, and pompano. **Note:** High cooking temperatures can destroy nearly half of these oils. It should also be remembered that only 1 tablespoon of fat is needed in the healthful daily diet, and that average Americans consume far more, often more than 6 or 8 tablespoons daily.

When purchasing fresh fish, promptly refrigerate it in its original wrapper. When preparing fish, cook it thoroughly, until the flesh is opaque throughout and separates when prodded with a fork. When selecting frozen fish, avoid any fishy odor, yellow discolorations, or ice crystals, which indicate a previous thawing.

Bonito Flakes Bonito flakes and dried shrimp powder are available in specialty sections or Mexican markets. Dried tuna and shrimp are available as tiny, dry flakes and have a highly concentrated flavor.

Haddock Related to the cod, this mild-flavored saltwater fish is replete with vitamin E, which helps to regulate both the vasomotor system and thyroid function in midlife women.

Mackerel This oily, savory fish from cold northern waters has valuable, highly unsaturated omega-3 fatty acids.

Fruit

Apples Apples are one of the top twenty-five vitamin E-bearing foods.

Apricots Fresh apricots are rich in vitamins C and E, while dried apricots have an abundance of vitamin A, which contributes to smoother, silkier midlife skin.

Blackberries Wild blackberries have a vitamin E content seven times greater than that of cultivated berries. Process carefully, as freezing destabilizes the vitamin.

Citrus Fruit Citrus fruit has a long history of efficacy in relieving menopausal symptoms, with much attention placed in recent years on a substance called limonene that occurs in oranges and lemons. Limonene boosts levels of naturally occurring enzymes in the body that are thought to break down carcinogens and stimulate cancer-killing immune cells. The rich brew of bioflavonoids found in citrus pulp and the thin white inner membrane of citrus fruits is full of vitamin-saturated estrogen substitutes, or phytoestrogens. As nutrients, bioflavonoids strengthen capillary walls, have a chemical activity similar to that of estrogen, and reduce the effects of hot flashes when consumed regularly. Identified by Dr. Susan Lark as the "menopause vitamin," bioflavonoids have shown dramatic curative results throughout the female system without any evidence of harmful effects.

Although estrogenic flavonoids are less potent than other plant estrogens—bioflavonoids have the same chemical structure as estrogen but 1/50,000th the strength—consumption of fruit pulp provides needed fiber as well as estrogenic activity. **A cooking tip:** Quickly pan-searing citrus with the membrane retains its fresh tang as well as preserves estrogenic properties.

Blood Orange This sweet-tart orange abounds in vitamin C, an all-important anti-stress vitamin. Its membrane contains phytoestrogenic bioflavonoids, which have properties similar to estrogen and work to relieve mood swings, anxiety, and irritability.

Grapes A delicious source of bioflavonoids, used to strengthen capillaries and regulate bleeding.

Mangoes Mangoes contain an ample supply of vitamin E, an antioxidant that strengthens capillaries, increases platelet movement, and protects against heart disease and arterial damage. Vitamin E improves blood cholesterol levels and, as an antioxidant, works to reverse age-related memory loss.

Look for mangoes with yellowish or red blushed skin, rather than deep green, and select the largest mangoes possible, since the hefty seed makes up much of the fruit's weight.

Papayas Silky smooth, with an exotic flavor and edible, peppery seeds, the papaya's rich store of vitamin A works to lessen skin conditions related to the aging process. Its stores of vitamin E help to alleviate premenstrual tension and breast cysts.

Peaches Dried peaches have an unusually high count of vitamin A, while fresh peaches also have stores of vitamin C, the anti-stress vitamin.

Grains

Whole grains, such as brown rice, corn, or barley, are complex carbohydrates, which, when broken down, help to stabilize blood sugar levels. Whole grains also contain vitamin E. Grains such as buckwheat and millet are high in fiber, and are also recommended for their magnesium content, while whole grains such as whole wheat, rye, and millet have both calcium and magnesium. The high oil content of grains means that they can become rancid quickly if not properly stored. Keep grains tightly sealed and stored in the refrigerator or freezer, and try to buy them in smaller amounts.

Herbs

Throughout history and across many cultures women have turned to herbs to alleviate menopausal distress, from night sweats and hot flashes to depression and fatigue. Ancient traditions are rich in such herbal decoctions, tinctures, and teas, yet to follow these recipes is to venture into nonstandard medicine, as yet anecdotal and largely clinically unproven. One of the largest health-care providers in the country has launched a comprehensive study of the effects of dong quai on menopausal symptoms; however, the final results will only be known after years of research. Without clinically controlled tests, we have only anecdotal history, established through years of application in naturopathy and various Eastern medicinal traditions and practices.

Since herbs are basically "medicines without prescription," doses should be minuscule and experimental—a half cup of tonic tea taken the first day, to make sure there is no adverse reaction.

Women who, because of personal medical history, must avoid estrogen supplements, should avoid ginseng, black cohosh, and dong quai (the female root of ginseng) because each contains estrogen-mimicking substances. Because of their estrogenic properties, teas made from these herbs should not be taken consistently.

Herbal Teas Hot-flash lore, based on the disturbance of hormonal rhythms, attributes a speeded-up metabolism to caffeine, hence higher body temperature and increased hot flashes. Coffee has also been associated with a rise in serum cholesterol. Why needle the system further? Moderate the day's caffeine quotient with herbal tea.

Not only do various herbs replace the body's estrogen, but they also boost the body's endocrine system to greater efficiency. Herbal teas are true pharmacopoeia, to be drunk in moderation—usually no more than 2 cups a day, depending on personal tolerance. Too much too fast may result in allergic reactions or, as in the case of ginseng, the steady accretion of estrogen, unbalanced by progesterone, resulting in a build-up of the lining of the uterine wall.

Preparation is important: Never brew teas or cook herbs in aluminum—always use glass or stainless steel pots. Take herbs on an empty stomach for best effect, and always 30 minutes to 2 hours before eating.

Culinary herbs can affect the body's circulation, hormonal balance, and digestion. They are antibiotic in nature, and are often deliciously flavored, a valuable addition to the daily midlife diet. Keep dried herbs in airtight containers. Do not oversteep teas—doing so can muddy or intensify a delicate flavor. For stronger tea, add more leaves at the beginning rather than oversteeping. An average tea strength is 1 tablespoon to 1 cup boiling water.

Asafetida A traditional Indian flavoring, usually in powdered form, made from the giant fennel root. Used in many Indian dishes as a garlic substitute. Available in Indian markets.

Blessed Thistle An herb taken for menopause fatigue, general run-down feelings, and depression.

Blue Vervain Another name for blue verbena, this herb was originally used by Native Americans to treat stomachaches and as a diuretic. Popular in herbal teas to fight hot flashes.

Cilantro Roots Both leaves and stem are tender enough for use in salads, while the root is used as a hot flash-reducing tea.

Cohosh, Black and Blue Black cohosh is used interchangeably with blue cohosh. Known medically for its sedative effect—due to the ingredient anemonin, which depresses the central nervous system—black cohosh is also considered an antispasmodic, used to relieve arthritis, muscle and nerve pain, even headaches and tinnitis. Its rhizomes and roots reportedly lower cholesterol levels, as well as lowering blood pressure and expanding blood vessels. Black cohosh was the standard birthing-room remedy for nineteenth-century women, who used it to regulate uterine contractions during labor. It was also the main ingredient of Lydia Pinkham's famed Vegetable Compound, quaffed by nineteenth-century women to relieve menstrual cramps.

Most noted for its estrogenlike action, cohosh is able to regulate and normalize hormone production, particularly during menopause. Composed of estrogenic substances, it offers quick herbal relief for unpleasant hot flashes.

> **CAUTION**
>
> *An overdose can result in dizziness, intense headaches, visual problems, slowed pulse, nausea, and vomiting. Use in moderation or with recommendations by experienced herbalists.*

The Hot Flash Cookbook

Dong Quai Noted for its strengthening and blood-building properties, this small whitish root of the lovage plant (a member of the carrot family), when used over an initial 6- to 8-week trial period, is a powerful uterine tonic approved by medical herbalists for menstrual irregularities. A gentle herb, generally believed to be estrogenic, it reputedly balances and moderates hormonal production, hence the term "adaptogenic." Its rich storehouse of phytoestrogens can stimulate the body's immune system into self-regulation. During menopause, dong quai helps to tone the reproductive organs, easing a woman through the hormonal shift. Long used by Chinese women—and available in Chinese pharmacies from Hong Kong to San Francisco in the form of Women's Precious Pills—it is known to strengthen female reproductive organs and reenergize the blood, while acting as an estrogen on the uterine and vaginal linings. The normal drop in the body's natural estrogen levels leaves the vaginal walls thin and dry. Estrogen, or an estrogen-mimicking substance, circulates in the bloodstream and acts on cells, plumping up the cell membranes and giving the walls more elasticity and strength.

Although noted for its "hot flash" relief properties, the adaptable qualities of dong quai allow it to work either way in the system, even performing as an antiestrogen, if necessary, countering the effects of estrogen. Similar in taste to its Western cousin, angelica, and available in thin dried slabs at natural foods stores, dong quai is rich in minerals, particularly iron. It can be grated, chopped, steeped, or steamed, as well as brewed as a tea. It has a uniquely strong, earthy taste that becomes too pungent with the slightest overcooking. An appropriate amount for most women is 2 teaspoons of the root twice a day.

> **CAUTION**
>
> *Teas, tinctures, or tonics containing ginseng, dong quai, and others such as black or blue cohosh should not be used during acute stages of illness or by those with chronic illness, including high blood pressure.*

False Unicorn Root Long cherished by women for its soothing effects on the female reproductive system, this root contains estrogenic precursors—hormonelike saponins—that help balance hormonal production and nourish the ovaries. Recognized by its gently bowed shape, the root is also known as "blazing star" and is distinguished from true unicorn root by its Latin name *Chamaelireum luteum*.

Ginseng This adaptogenic herb stimulates the body's immune system to encourage self-regulation and is useful for the treatment of hot flashes. Ginseng is widely used throughout different world cultures to boost energy levels. Of the myriad types of ginseng available, two are used most widely. Although Siberian ginseng has been discovered only recently, it is considered by many to be the safest for long-term use. For menopausal women, it may combat fatigue by helping the body adapt to stress—arguably, by improving the function of the adrenal glands. Used by long-distance runners in the former Soviet Union to achieve greater endurance, ginseng can also reverse menopausal depression, debility, fatigue, and stress in midlife women. The other type of ginseng, panax, is native to China and derives its strength as a sexual energizer from a group of compounds called ginsenosides. It contains approximately eleven hormonelike saponins that exert adaptogenic, or stress-protective, properties. When taken daily, ginseng will normalize the body's response to temperature changes.

In China, ginseng is usually combined with, and tamed by, herbs such as licorice. Asians consider ginseng an effective tonic for the elderly. A third type, American ginseng, has similar rejuvenative qualities.

Licorice Root Containing a wealth of vitamins, including vitamin E, licorice decoctions have an estrogenlike hormonal effect that stimulates adrenal gland function, and also decreases muscle spasms. So widely used for its calming effect it is called the "peacemaker" in China, licorice, or "sweet root," is recognized throughout Asia for its soothing effect on menopausal discomfort.

How much licorice is too much? Taken in high doses for a long period of time, licorice is used in Asian cultures as an energy tonic and to boost immunity, increase estrogen levels, and strengthen the cardiovascular system. Also used as a candy flavor, licorice may cause swelling and a salt imbalance, which will vanish as soon as use is discontinued. Generally considered mild and nontoxic, licorice still poses a risk for those with high blood pressure, although the recorded cases of high blood pressure and water retention came from using highly concentrated extracts, rather than the whole herb.

Mint Mint has long been used to aid digestion, hurry childbirth, cleanse wounds, and even to wash cheese to prevent decay. Native Americans roasted and salted the leaves, or boiled them as an infusion to dispel fevers or cure respiratory problems. Coupled with licorice, mint decreases fatigue. Sip mint tea in moderation at first, building to a daily cup or two, no more.

Mirin A sweet wine used for Japanese sauces and glazes. Also called rice wine or sweet sake. Substitute dry sherry.

Miso Paste A fermented soy product, originally from Japan, with a much lower salt content than regular salt. Ideal for flavoring soups and rice dishes, it has high amounts of B vitamins and protein. Keep refrigerated in an airtight container.

Sarsaparilla Jamaican sarsaparilla has the greatest herbal concentration of natural progesterone, considered by many health care practitioners to be a valuable counterpart to natural estrogen in maintaining a healthy, natural balance. Its North American counterpart, also called wild ginseng, wild licorice, rabbit root, or small spikenard, was used by Native Americans to make a sweat-inducing tea believed to alleviate rheumatism, gout, and skin diseases. They subsisted on the root for days during war excursions. They also chewed the roots to make a poultice. Its root provides the tea commonly used for menopause, a refreshing brew with a bitter licorice flavor. The reddish-brown color is redolent of the turn-of-the-century drink, sarsaparilla.

Old herbal books list this aromatic root as a healing base for diseases of the blood, chronic rheumatism, "cardiology, bellyache, etc." In addition, as a syrup it was used to treat scrofula and other skin diseases. The fresh root was used for fainting and fits, pounded and made into a poultice, and even brewed into a tea in which gill nets were soaked before being set out to catch fish for the night.

Nuts

The Brazil nut is really a seed and the peanut a legume, yet they join a host of bonafide nutmeats that harbor vitamin E as well as a preponderance of mono-saturated "good" fat. Nut profiles can vary. The almond is an excellent fiber source, low in sodium, high in folate and zinc, and a good source of magnesium, which helps regulate blood pressure and hot flashes. Some nuts, like the Brazil nut, are high in fats, but they also contain healthful compounds such as ellagic acid, which seems to eliminate certain cancer-causing agents from the body. Almonds, hazelnuts, and walnuts contain the highest amount of vitamin E. Nuts should be purchased in modest amounts and stored in airtight containers, because they go rancid easily due to their high oil content.

Hazelnuts Hazelnuts are delicious when used in soups and salad dressings. Polyunsaturated hazelnut oil must be kept cold to maintain its fresh and distinctive taste. Both oil and nuts are high in vitamin E, an essential antioxidant that protects cells from breakdown.

Toasting and Peeling Hazelnuts Preheat oven to 350°F. Spread the nuts on a baking sheet and bake for about 10 minutes, or until toasted. Wrap the nuts in a towel and let steam for 1 minute. Rub the nuts with the towel to remove the skin, then cool.

Peanuts Peanuts are actually legumes, not nuts, that contain essential magnesium to lower blood pressure, lower colesterol, reduce platelet clogging to assist the heart, and restore the body's vital ability to absorb calcium.

Toasting Nuts Preheat the oven to 375°F. Spread the nuts on a baking sheet. Place in the oven for 3 to 5 minutes, or until lightly toasted. Turn the nuts occasionally with a spatula, or shake the pan or sheet, making sure the nuts don't slide off.

Oils

When sautéeing in oil, wait just until the oil begins to smoke and a slight ripple appears on its surface. A moment too long, and overheating results, with a loss of valuable vitamin E.

Canola Oil Contains plenty of vitamin E to combat hot flashes, anxiety, and irritation. Canola oil is a preferred monosaturated vegetable oil that has not been heat-extracted and is free of unhealthy fatty acids. Look for organic, expeller-pressed canola oil at natural foods stores.

Hazelnut Oil Polyunsaturated hazelnut oil must be kept cold to maintain its fresh but distinct taste. Use in soups and salad dressings. Both oil and nuts are high in vitamin E, an essential antioxidant that protects cells from breakdown.

Olive Oil Olive oil, a rich food source of vitamin E, reduces premenstrual tension and menopausal mood swings. Store large amounts in the refrigerator.

Sesame Oil A household mainstay in China for 5,000 years, Asian sesame oil is a dark, strongly flavored oil made from toasted sesame seeds. A nutty-flavored, light sesame oil made from untoasted seeds is also available. Both have a stable shelf life, lend sparkle to a fried or sautéed dish, and are full of essential fats and heart-protecting vitamin E.

Wheat Germ Oil Wheat germ oil, rich in vitamin E, works to stabilize hormonal swings, ease fatigue, and also to smooth and plump the skin.

Poultry and Meats

Centerpiece or seasoning? The question of how much meat is too much often defines the difference between an affluent lifestyle and that of traditional cultures. Studies comparing cholesterol levels point to the efficacy of carbohydrates and plant protein rather than animal fats. Experts agree that saturated fats should make up less than 10 percent of caloric intake.

Choose organic meat whenever possible. Some cows and chickens are fed or implanted with synthetic growth hormones. These hormones are forms of estrogen and are known to cause runaway cell growth that may lead to cancer.

Lamb Vitamin E-bearing foods, such as lamb and leeks, may reduce free-radical levels in the blood, thus slowing down cell oxidation and stress.

Seeds

Extremely high in digestible calcium, seeds are an ideal part of a bone-enhancement diet. Nutritionists have suggested that sesame seeds should be toasted, then ground for better digestibility—several seconds in a blender does the task.

Aniseed Gives a sweet, licorice flavor that enhances pastries, sauces, and vegetables. Also delicious in herbal teas as a plant source of estrogen. Used traditionally to quell hot flashes.

Fennel Seeds Crisp cleansers of the palate after a flavorful meal, fennel seeds are as traditional in parts of Asia and India as the after-dinner mint in the West. The aromatic oils in the seeds aid digestive juices.

Flaxseed Particularly rich in phytoestrogens, the shiny luster and luscious texture of flaxseeds are part of an almost-oily presentation. In the mouth, flaxseeds slide and slither, making them easier to eat if baked into a dish, ground up, or pureed. They are a rich source of essential omega-3 fatty acids, particularly when taken as oil. Flaxseed oil loses its nutritive value when heated; always use at room temperature, or even chilled. The efficacy of the omega-3 is further ensured by taking a small amount of vitamin B-6 as well as a protein containing sulfur, such as low-fat cottage cheese.

Sesame Seeds Sesame seeds are rich in vitamin E, with estrogenlike properties that act as an antioxidant, protecting cells and tissues from some of the visible effects of aging.

Toasting Seeds Heat a dry skillet over high heat. Pour the seeds into the hot pan, shaking to turn. Toast for 3 to 5 minutes, or until slightly brown.

Spices

Cayenne Pepper Contains high levels of magnesium and bioflavonoids, nutrients essential to the relief of hot flashes, fatigue, and depression. Ironically, this extremely hot and pungent pepper, grown in Mexico and Guatemala, effectively quells hot flash symptoms when used in moderation.

Ginger Ginger is a crossover spice in many cultures, starring in both the culinary and medicinal world. Warming and stimulating, long used in Chinese medicine for its tonic effects, ginger is also used to aid digestion, rid the tired system of fatigue and weakness, and as a natural cleansing and purifying agent. From hot beverage to candied condiment, the pungent, piquant zing of ginger has been called an aphrodisiac as well as a palliative to indigestion, neutralizing offensive elements in other foods that produce indigestion. In addition, ginger was an antidote for pregnancy-related ills such as morning sickness, aiding in fighting off nausea. Candied ginger was a household sweet in medieval and Tudor times, used to counteract the rank gaminess of poultry and the odor of fish. Ginger mixed in wine was also believed to prevent the plague.

Today, ginger speeds and assists the digestion of proteins, can prevent motion sickness, fights intestinal parasites, and protects against ulcers. It is excellent in combating fatigue, inertia, and depression. Its chemistry is complex; dried ginger is more useful as an anti-inflammatory and has decidedly more analgesic effects than grated fresh root ginger. Unlike some over-the-counter anti-inflammatory drugs, ginger protects the lining of the stomach, according to Dr. Andrew Weil. Either fresh or dried, ginger is a peppy tonic that spurs the circulatory system to renewed vigor.

Ginger root is a storehouse of iron, particularly good for chronic fatigue, headaches, low energy, or irritability. Although hot and fiery, ginger also has soothing traces of calcium, which is helpful in the effort to reverse bone loss in osteoporosis. It is high in calories and sodium (crystallized) and has a little fat.

Although called a root, it is an underground stem, or rhizome, that can sprout new roots and shoots.

Look for young, fresh ginger, identified by its smooth, taut, wrinkle-free skin. The brightest flavor comes from the young, pinkish "fingers" of baby ginger, but both baby and regular ginger are power-packed with iron and are effective against chronic fatigue, headaches, low energy, or irritability. Ginger maintains its crispness for weeks if wrapped in a paper towel, stored in an airtight plastic container, and placed in the warmer part of the refrigerator. Do not freeze ginger. It will soften, shrivel, and turn to mush. You can also store sliced fresh ginger for up to six months in a container with a favorite liquor, such as sherry, gin, or vodka.

Tofu

Soy products are easy to digest, are an excellent source of vegetable protein, and are rich in phytoestrogens. Mounting evidence shows that soybean phytoestrogens alleviate the side effects of menopause. Perhaps this is the reason why Japanese women complain of fewer hot flashes than their American counterparts. "Asian women eat hundreds of times more phytoestrogens than American women," according to Kaiser endocrinologist Dr. Bruce Ettinger, to which he attributes their longer menstrual cycles, fewer heart attacks, and a lower risk of breast cancer.

How does the soybean affect hot flashes? The longer menstrual cycles triggered in premenopausal women by daily servings of soy protein suggest an estrogenlike effect. This has been borne out by several as yet unpublished studies on soy isoflavones.

Isoflavones are estrogen look-alikes found in tofu that strongly resemble a woman's own hormones and quell the occurrence of hot flashes and night sweats. Most soy isoflavones are far weaker than human estrogen, about one thousandth the potency. A study reported by the American Dietetic Association in 1995 compared the use of fermented soy products versus unfermented, with results suggesting that fermentation increases the availability of isoflavones in soy.

The exact ratio of soy to estrogen, or the amount of soy needed to act as an estrogen source, is still unknown, but its other salubrious effects have been proven:

a mere 25 grams of soy protein lowers cholesterol, while 1½ cups of tofu daily reduces the risk of certain types of cancer. The particular form of isoflavones found in soy, called genistein, is a potent antioxidant, flushing unstable oxygen molecules from the body before they have the chance to turn cancerous. Research reveals that 5 to 6 ounces of firm tofu daily lowers LDL cholesterol, as well as provides a blend of phytochemicals that may play a role in disease prevention. As a plant protein, soy is rich in soluble fiber. In Japan, where tofu is almost always on the table, breast cancer is four times less common than in the United States.

Soybeans offer the highest-quality protein of any plant food, containing all eight essential amino acids, as well as a host of phytochemicals.

Miso, made of cooked aged soybeans, has a salty flavor that is delicious in soups. It comes in several varieties, including white and red.

Tempeh, a food that originated on the island of Java perhaps as long as a thousand years ago, derives its name from an Indonesian word for fermented foods, and is the only soy dish not to originate in China or Japan. To prepare tempeh, cooked soybeans are well drained, exposed to spores, packed in aerated containers, and incubated for twenty-four hours, or until the beans are tightly bound together. The soybeans are often blended with rice or grains, then fermented. After cooking and fermentation, the protein is more available and the natural sugars are reduced, making it easily digestible. Soy tempeh is protein-rich, containing 19.5 percent protein compared to 17.9 percent protein for hamburger. In stores, it is available in a firm, ready-to-cook, molded form that can be fried, baked, or steamed. Fried tempeh is cited as the most meatlike in flavor and texture. Tempeh often has a sprinkling of black spots or dark mold, which only means that the "good" bacteria are still at work.

NOTE

Soy is a useful and versatile protein and nondairy calcium source, nourishing to nearly everyone, but high in salt content. Those taking synthetic thyroid hormones should limit soy products because of their thyroid-blocking capability.

Hot Flash Foods

Vegetables

Every mouthful of a nutritious leafy green vegetable is chockful of vitamins, especially vitamin E. In addition, leafy greens go beyond the realm of "hot flash control" by virtue of their high calcium content, thereby offering double and even triple advantages to the midlife woman.

As a protection against hypertension, calcium, when complemented by magnesium, relieves muscle spasms and cramping by inhibiting the production of lactic acid, which causes muscle soreness and pain. It also replenishes the gradual leaching of calcium from the bones, which occurs during and after menopause. Although not directly able to affect hot flashes, calcium is closely linked to estrogen, and plays a major role in the prevention of osteoporosis. Estrogen helps improve the absorption of calcium, which helps to harden bones. Both are found in vegetables as well as dairy products. Today's emphasis on lowering daily fat intake encourages a more vegan approach to dietary choices.

Quite simply, an aging body, no matter how well exercised or nutritionally fit, cannot accommodate a milk-related arterial buildup of cholesterol or plaque. Drinking whole milk can create, quite literally, a blockage, as the fat-laden particles refuse to pass through the cell membrane. Whole milk is high in fat, low in complex carbohydrates and fiber—even its bonus amounts of calcium, when laced with fat, *deplete* the body's stored reserves of calcium rather than aid in replenishment. Fat interferes with the absorption of magnesium, which is the key ingredient for strong bones; therefore any cause of a magnesium imbalance is a subtle threat to solid bones.

Vegetables can serve as a healthful and substantive dairy alternative; 1 cup of cooked kale has more calcium than 1 cup of milk, as well as provides direct "hot flash" intervention with its stores of vitamin E. Broccoli, collard greens, dandelions, mustard greens, chickweed, kale, chard, and wild oats are calcium-rich, easy to prepare, and virtually fat-free foods readily available at natural foods stores.

Asparagus Rich in vitamin E, this popular vegetable, when lightly steamed, preserves the estrogenlike characteristics of vitamin E, a nutrient that lulls the overstressed system and banishes fatigue.

Avocado The avocado abounds in potassium, which helps balance body fluids and eases menopause fatigue. Its vitamin E content offers vasomotor support and quells hot flashes.

Beans, Dried Rich in calcium and potassium, which prompt surges of energy. Fights menopausal fatigue.

Beet Greens Cooked beet greens abound in vitamin C and vitamin E, an important antioxidant. Vitamin C revitalizes, as well as helps control erratic bleeding. Leafy greens also have a high calcium content.

Bell Peppers, Red Red peppers have far more international units of vitamin A than most other vegetables, which helps to prevent age-related skin conditions.

   Roasting and Peeling Peppers and Chiles Roast the peppers or chiles over an open gas flame or roast in 450°F oven until the skin darkens and blisters. Place the peppers or chiles in a closed paper bag and let sit for about 20 minutes. Peel the peppers or chiles and remove the seeds and stem.

Broccoli Extremely rich in vitamin A, which helps midlife skin conditions and spotty bleeding. Also contains vitamin E, to combat hot flashes and osteoarthritis and contains a recently identified substance, sulphoraphane—a powerful cancer preventative. Broccoli's outer leaf is the most vitamin-rich part of the plant.

Cabbage A food source of calcium, which soothes anxiety by relieving symptoms of hypertension.

Carrot Leaves Vitamin E concentrates in the leaves of the carrot. E is noted for its ability to ease tension, soothe skin conditions, and protect cells from oxidation.

Celery Leaves Vitamin E is saturated in the outer leaves of the celery stalk, which was once used as a medicinal herb.

Dandelion Greens One of the richest green leafy vegetables, abounding in vitamin A and calcium, which helps stabilize the constant leaching from the bones.

Fennel Brewed as tea, eaten raw, and cooked as a bulb, this lightly scented, crunchy Mediterranean favorite offers up estrogenic hormonal activity and is the subject of much new research. Often seen growing wild in pastures and fields as well as for sale in supermarkets, sweet anise or, in Italian, *finocchio*, sports a feathery crown of aromatic leaves that wave over its celerylike stalks. The seeds crackle with the flavor of licorice herbal tea, and the deep green fronds offer an aromatic bed for meats or seafood, or a lively savor when chopped and sprinkled over pasta dishes. Eaten raw, fennel has a bright but cool flavor of anise; baked or broiled, the licorice taste grows densely sweet and rich, and honors this vegetable's centuries-old reputation as a salubrious herbal panacea. The Roman naturalist Pliny identified numerous remedies using fennel. Today, it is prescribed world-wide as an appetite and dieting aid. Lightly toasted, crunchy, and refreshing fennel seeds are used in Asia as a digestive aid—their aromatic oils are believed to stimulate the flow of digestive juices. Used as a tea (1 cup boiling water to 1 teaspoon of fennel seeds, covered and steeped for 10 minutes), the seeds both warm and stimulate. Adding dried fennel twigs to a charcoal or wood fire is a common Provençal method of cooking fish; the fennel bed imparts a clean flavor to fish.

Garlic Garlic use is legendary, from rubbing it on cuts and abrasions, to preventing infections, to curing colds. It acts to lower the body's blood sugar, and reduce menopausal fatigue and weakness. Garlic also works to moderate hypertension, if consumed regularly.

Hijiki A sea vegetable that helps to maintain bone density and inhibit the steady demineralization and leaching of calcium.

Kale The superabundance of vitamin A in kale helps to ease environmental stresses and contributes to heart health. Vitamin E helps to strengthen capillary walls and, when taken regularly, reduces the effects of hot flashes. Kale is rich in calcium and iron, as well as the antioxidant vitamin E. Kale's estrogenlike properties work to provide relief for menopausal mood swings.

Mustard Greens High in calcium, which, when complemented by magnesium, relieves muscle spasms and cramping by inhibiting the production of lactic acid. Greens also replenish calcium loss from the bones.

Sorrel Be sure to discard any leaves that are limp or discolored, since crisp, green vegetation not only releases a stronger flavor but more nutrients.

Wakame Rich in vitamin E, this sea vegetable has a delicately flavored dark green leaf. When rinsed in cold water and soaked for 15 minutes, wakame makes a delicious addition to soups and dressings, or use as a garnish for fish.

Watercress Watercress is loaded with bone-building calcium and makes a savory addition to salads.

Yams Dense and sweet as life itself, the flesh of this member of the morning glory family counts among its essential ingredients a host of workaday plant steroids essential to the production of both progesterone and vitamin E. Popular in folk medicine for centuries and more recently in the Western scientific community, the yam is both delicious and efficacious. The most advanced research in hormonal activity has been conducted with *Dioscorea villosa,* the wild Mexican yam. Long used by herbalists, today the Mexican yam is widely used throughout the world. It contains diosgenin, which is easily converted to natural progesterone and is the basis for estrogen and progesterone synthesis.

The yam suffers an identification problem in this country. The "yams" available in the United States are actually sweet potatoes and, as such, do not possess the natural progesterone of the Mexican yam. The tubers marketed as "yams" are the deep red Garnet or the bright orange, coppery-hued Jewel, which are really yamlike potatoes. While they lack phytoestrogens, they do have an abundance of vitamin E.

Those interested in obtaining wild Mexican yams, or their Nigerian counterparts, will find them advertised over the Internet both as tubers and as seeds, or in specialty ethnic markets, but they are rare. Do not plan a dinner menu around them.

FOODS TO MINIMIZE OR AVOID

Before embarking on a healthy new regimen, there are a few foods to consider minimizing. Many of these foods aggravate undesirable symptoms and do not promote a healthy diet.

Alcohol

Not only does alcohol dehydrate the skin, which adds to unsightly dryness and wrinkling, but it is known to lengthen the duration of hot flashes and add to their severity. Although small amounts can be relaxing (according to Dr. Susan Lark, 4 ounces of wine per day, 10 ounces of beer, and 1 ounce of hard liquor), anything more should be taken with caution.

Butter

Despite the fact that butter appears in some recipes in this book, its high fat content makes it unacceptable for frequent use. Substitute any of the delicious vegetable oils.

Coffee

No single elixir has insinuated itself into our lives as has coffee. It has the reliable effect of providing a predictable jolt of energy that kick-starts our day, along with a startling ability to throw the midlife woman into an immediate hot flash. For those who will not forego their morning cup, its effects can be buffered with low-fat milk and by sipping it slowly rather than gulping it down. This can lessen the force of major flashes to that of light "flash" temblors. However, the inescapable truth is that coffee triggers hot flashes, particularly in the first months and/or years of menopause.

Coffee use can be moderated or completely replaced by herbal drinks, hot broths, vegetable waters, and grain-based substitutes such as Postum. Not all women will enjoy Postum, even though a cup, if substituted for coffee, saves the beleaguered bones from the calcium drain of caffeine. Each cup of coffee robs the body of 11 milligrams of calcium. Lack of exercise also makes it difficult for the body to absorb calcium, and a high-protein diet depletes the body of calcium.

Salt

Salt is a particularly virulent hot-flash trigger, and should be relinquished in favor of other flavorings such as miso, commercial nonsodium seasonings, and herbs such as basil, tarragon, and oregano. Sodium chloride has been linked to heart hypertension.

Spices

Avoiding the more stressful spices, such as black pepper and salt, leaves a host of mild yet flavorful seasonings with which to enhance food: dill, thyme, cinnamon, and sage, to name a few. Some spices, such as cayenne, are rich in magnesium and potassium, which provide hot-flash relief as well as lessening other menopausal symptoms.

Sugar

Refined sugar also triggers sweats and jitters, but is easily replaced by fruit juice concentrates, minced dried fruits, or dried fruits softened in hot water and pureed.

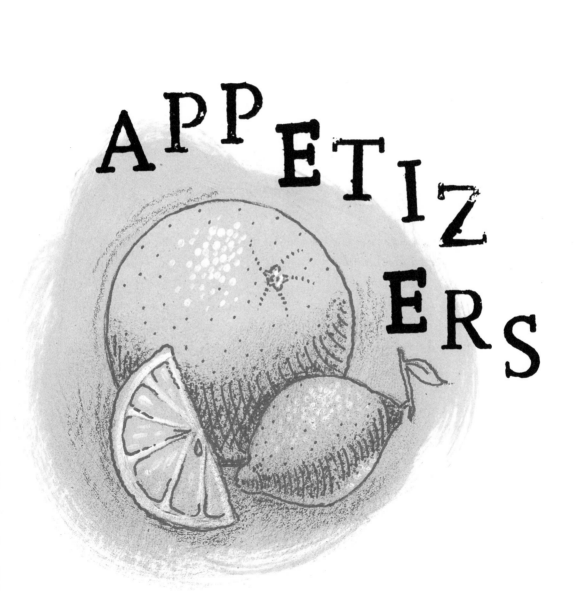

APPETIZERS

Asparagus
With Sesame Dip

Makes 6 servings

This dish provides a mouth-pleasing sensation of crisp and crunch, plus dipping ease. Lightly steamed stalks are dipped in soy and vinegar, then in toasted sesame.

1 bunch thin asparagus, trimmed

½ cup low-salt soy sauce

½ cup plain rice vinegar

1 cup sesame seeds, toasted (see page 55)

In a covered steamer or saucepan, steam the asparagus over boiling water until crisp-tender, about 5 minutes. Plunge them into cold water and drain. Fan out on a large serving platter.

Mix the soy sauce and rice vinegar together in a small bowl and serve cold alongside the asparagus. Place the sesame seeds in another bowl.

Have guests dip each asparagus spear in the soy sauce, then into the sesame seeds.

TOASTED SESAME
AND SPINACH BALLS

Makes 2 to 4 servings

This spirited combination invokes centuries of Japanese culinary tradition as well as exclamations of delight. Sesame-coated inky-green spinach balls are attractive appetizers.

1 bunch fresh spinach, chard, or kale, stemmed

¼ cup sesame seeds, toasted (see page 55)

¼ cup plain rice vinegar

2 tablespoons low-salt soy sauce

Pinch of grated fresh ginger

If using kale, trim the leaves away from the thick stem. In a covered steamer or saucepan, steam the leaves over boiling water for 2 minutes, or until limp. Let cool, then squeeze the moisture from the leaves and press them into balls. Roll each ball in the toasted sesame seeds. Mix the vinegar, soy sauce, and ginger in a small bowl. Drizzle the dressing over the balls just before serving.

ASPARAGUS
WITH FENNEL CURLS

Makes 4 servings

This dish, rich in vitamin E, makes a forthright presentation.
Bright green stalks are laced with airy fennel curls and tiny, crisp
garlic slivers.

2 fennel stalks

¼ cup extra-virgin olive oil

1 pound asparagus, trimmed

6 garlic cloves, minced

With a thin, sharp knife, cut the fennel stalks along the grain until a thin
"ribbon" of fennel curls up. Leave the ribbons in long strands, loop for a
bird's-nest effect, or cut in half for shorter curls. Set aside.

In a large skillet or sauté pan over high heat, heat the oil and sauté the
asparagus for 5 minutes. Add the garlic and cook for 1 minute. Serve at once,
garnished with the shaved fennel curls.

Black Bean
AND TOFU RELISH

Makes about 3 cups

This lively relish is a postmodern flavor experience that mingles the traditional flavors of East and West. Serve with steamed vegetables, or as a topping for potatoes, pizza, or crisp tortillas. Rich in viamin E.

1 teaspoon soybean oil

1 shallot, minced

3 garlic cloves, minced

1 Anaheim chile, roasted, peeled, and diced (see page 59)

2 bell peppers, roasted, peeled, and diced (see page 59)

¼ cup plain rice vinegar

1 teaspoon cumin seeds, toasted and crushed (see page 55)

¼ teaspoon fenugreek seeds, toasted and crushed (see page 55)

½ teaspoon grated lime zest

Salt and freshly ground pepper to taste

10 ounces firm tofu, rinsed and drained

1½ cups cooked black beans, drained

3 tablespoons minced fresh cilantro

In a medium sauté pan or skillet, heat the oil over medium-high heat. Add the shallot and garlic and sauté until translucent, about 1 minute. Add the chile, peppers, and vinegar and bring to a boil. Remove from heat and add the cumin, fenugreek, zest, salt, and pepper. Stir to combine and set aside.

In a large bowl, mash the tofu, then add the beans and mix thoroughly. Add the cilantro and the vinegar mixture; toss to combine. Let cool before serving or refrigerate overnight.

Appetizers

Power Dose Orange Sauté

Makes 4 servings

This unusual combination, based on delicate Valencia oranges with paper-thin skins, has a range of bioflavonoid activity enhanced by a peppery dash of cayenne. Quick-cooking retains maximum estrogenic properties.

2 unpeeled Valencia oranges

½ yellow onion

1 tomato

1 tablespoon extra-virgin olive oil

2 garlic cloves, minced

2 tablespoons balsamic vinegar

Salt and freshly ground pepper to taste

⅛ teaspoon cayenne pepper

⅛ teaspoon sugar

Pita bread for serving

With a very sharp knife, cut the oranges, onion, and tomato into wafer-thin crosswise slices. In a sauté pan, over high heat, heat the olive oil and sauté the oranges, onion, tomato, and garlic. Sauté for 2 to 4 minutes, or until the oranges are beginning to brown.

In a small bowl, whisk together all the remaining ingredients except the pita bread.

Arrange the orange mixture on a platter. Drizzle with the balsamic mixture. Serve at once with pita bread.

SOUTHWEST CHILE-TOFU DIP

Makes 3 cups

A creamy tofu base turns *picante* and picks up the vivid flavors and colors of the Southwest. A bright flower garnish will contrast nicely with its deep reddish hue.

1 red bell pepper, roasted, peeled, and sliced (see page 59)

2 large garlic cloves, minced

1 tablespoon grated fresh ginger

4 scallions, white and green parts separated and finely chopped

1 Anaheim chile, seeded and minced

1 jalapeño chile, seeded and minced

2 pounds soft tofu, rinsed and drained

⅓ cup soy sauce

¼ cup plain rice vinegar

2 tablespoons Asian sesame oil

4 teaspoons honey or sugar, or to taste

Freshly ground pepper to taste

2 to 4 tablespoons low-salt vegetable broth or water

Nonfat tortilla chips for serving

In a medium bowl, combine the red pepper, garlic, ginger, and white part of the scallions. Transfer to a blender or food processor and add all the remaining ingredients except the green scallions, broth or water, and chips. Puree until smooth, adding broth or water as needed.

Transfer to a bowl. Cover and let sit for at least 1 hour. Sprinkle with chopped green scallions. Serve with tortilla chips.

Spicy Tofu and Tomato Dip

Makes 8 servings

Serve this dip, by Linda Hillel, with celery sticks and thin slices of baguette.

2 tomatoes, seeded and cut into chunks

2 scallions, green parts only, thinly sliced

One 10-ounce package soft tofu,
   rinsed and drained

2 garlic cloves, pressed

2 tablespoons extra-virgin olive oil

2 teaspoons balsamic vinegar

½ teaspoon red pepper flakes

1 tablespoon minced fresh marjoram
   or oregano, or 1 teaspoon dried

Kosher salt and freshly ground pepper to taste

Chop the tomatoes and scallions in a blender or food processor until thoroughly mixed. Add the remaining ingredients and puree until smooth.

GREEN RICE CUBES

Makes 8 cubes

These vitamin-packed squares of spinach and rice are unusual but so easy to make. In place of soy sauce, drizzle with a favorite curry or satay sauce.

6 ounces spinach, stemmed and finely chopped

3½ cups water

2 cups long-grain white rice

Salt and freshly ground pepper to taste

Low-salt soy sauce for drizzling

In a covered steamer or saucepan, steam the spinach over boiling water until limp, about 3 minutes. Transfer to a blender or food processor and puree until smooth. Set aside.

Combine the water and rice in a large pan. Cover and bring to a boil; reduce heat and cook until the water is absorbed, about 25 minutes. Stir in the spinach puree and cook for 5 minutes. Add salt and pepper.

Spoon the hot rice into an oiled 10-inch square pan, pressing it firmly into the pan with a spoon. Rinse the spoon with water as needed to prevent the rice from sticking. Let the rice cool completely. Run a knife around the pan edge, then turn the rice out onto a cutting board. Cut into 1-inch cubes with a knife, rinsing the knife in cold water after each cut. Arrange the cubes on a platter and drizzle with a little soy sauce.

Sun-dried Tomato and Tofu Pâté

Makes 6 servings

Made with firm tofu, this pâté by Linda Hillel can be used as a sandwich filling with lettuce or sprouts, and it excels as an appetizer when paired with toasted sourdough bread or crackers.

⅓ cup oil-packed sun-dried tomatoes
    with a little of the oil

½ cup packed fresh basil leaves

2 garlic cloves, pressed

14 ounces firm tofu, rinsed and drained

2 tablespoons balsamic vinegar

Kosher salt and freshly ground pepper to taste

2 tablespoons pine nuts, toasted
    (see page 52)

In a blender or food processor, puree the sun-dried tomatoes, basil, and garlic until smooth. Add all the remaining ingredients. Puree briefly for a chunky pâté, longer for a smoother texture.

MARINATED TOFU CUBES WITH HERBS

Makes 6 to 8 servings

Served with crudités of fennel, celery, carrots, and jicama, these bouncy squares, created by Linda Hillel, are delightfully chewable, zestfully phytoactive, and deeply flavored.

2 tablespoons Dijon mustard

Dash of cayenne pepper

1 garlic clove, halved

¼ cup minced fresh herbs: any combination of parsley, basil, tarragon, thyme, chives, and/or dill

1 teaspoon dried rosemary, marjoram, or oregano (or a combination)

¼ cup oil-packed sun-dried tomatoes, slivered

¼ cup balsamic vinegar

¼ cup extra-virgin olive oil

Kosher salt and freshly ground pepper to taste

14 ounces firm tofu, rinsed, drained, and patted dry

In a medium bowl, whisk together all the ingredients except the tofu and set aside.

Cut the tofu into ½-inch cubes. Place in a nonaluminum container, drizzle with the marinade, cover tightly, and refrigerate overnight or up to several days. Gently shake the container occasionally to turn the tofu in the marinade. Serve at room temperature with toothpicks for spearing.

Appetizers

Cold Ginger Tofu

Makes 8 servings

Creamy as custard but firm enough for skewering, cool tofu cubes are a natural match for hot ginger. In this recipe by Linda Hillel, the tofu cubes glisten in a pool of spicy sauce.

10 ounces firm tofu, rinsed, drained, and patted dry

½ cup slivered shiso or thinly sliced scallions

¼ cup low-salt soy sauce

3 tablespoons grated fresh ginger

¼ cup dried bonito flakes, or 2 tablespoons shrimp powder (available in Asian markets)

Fresh mint sprigs for garnish

Cut the tofu into ½-inch cubes and arrange on a plate. Sprinkle with the shiso or scallions.

Whisk together the soy sauce and ginger and drizzle over the tofu. Sprinkle with bonito flakes or shrimp powder. Skewer with toothpicks and garnish with mint.

SWEET MILLET CROQUETTES
WITH GINGER-NUT CHUTNEY

Makes about 16 croquettes

This "birdseed" grain is often supplanted by its more popular relatives, bulgur, cracked wheat, or rice. Yet millet commands its own attention in these dome-shaped delicacies, toasty brown and served with a thick chutney.

2½ cups water

¼ teaspoon salt

1 cup millet, thoroughly rinsed

1 sweet potato, peeled and cut into ¼-inch dice

5 scallions, finely chopped

Canola oil for brushing

Minced fresh cilantro for garnish

Ginger-Nut Chutney (recipe follows)

To make the croquettes: Preheat the oven to 400°F. Bring the water and salt to boil in a medium saucepan. Add the millet, lower heat, cover, and simmer for 10 minutes. Lay the sweet potato dice on top of the cooking millet without stirring. Cover and cook for 10 minutes. Transfer to a large bowl and let cool to the touch. Add the scallions and toss. The mixture should be sticky enough to hold its shape when formed into patties. Using ¼ cup mixture for each croquette, gently shape into ovals. Place on a baking sheet and brush with oil. Bake for 20 minutes, or until brown.

Sprinkle with cilantro and serve with the chutney.

Appetizers

GINGER-NUT CHUTNEY

Makes ¾ cup

½ cup roasted peanuts

Juice of 1 lemon

1 tablespoon minced fresh ginger

1 green onion, including the green part,
   finely chopped

1 garlic clove, minced

Place the peanuts and lemon juice in a blender or food processor, pulsing quickly to grind. Add the remaining ingredients and pulse into a paste.

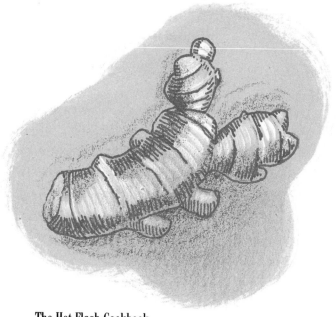

The Hot Flash Cookbook

Toasted Sunflower
Black Bean Tostadas

Makes 6 appetizers

An open gas flame gives an authentic smoky quality to tortillas topped with a spicy mix of black beans, nuts, and seeds.

1 cup cooked black beans, drained

¼ cup sunflower seeds, toasted

¼ cup toasted peanuts, crushed

Hot chili sauce to taste

Salt and cayenne pepper to taste

1 tomato, seeded and chopped

1 teaspoon ground cumin

1 celery stalk with leaves, finely chopped

2 tablespoons yogurt or sour cream

6 corn tortillas

In a medium bowl, thoroughly combine all the ingredients except the tortillas. Toast the tortillas by placing them, one at a time, over an open gas flame for 30 seconds, or until crisp, turning once or twice. Or, bake the tortillas directly on the oven racks of a preheated 450°F oven until crisp. Spread the topping on the toasted tortillas.

Hijiki Crab Cakes

Makes 8 servings

Use the outer leaves of green cabbage to show off the dramatic black tones of hijiki, a seaweed available in natural foods stores that tastes faintly of licorice.

5 ounces hijiki

¼ cup oil

1 pound fresh, lump crabmeat

1 red bell pepper, seeded, deribbed, and finely chopped

6 fresh white bread slices, crusts removed

1 tablespoon minced garlic

1 jalapeño chile, seeded and minced

2 tablespoons cilantro

1 whole outer cabbage leaf, minced

2 tablespoons filé powder or seafood seasoning

Salt and freshly ground pepper to taste

SAUCE   ¼ cup mayonnaise

¼ cup prepared horseradish

Rinse the hijiki to remove sand and debris, then soak in water to cover for 10 minutes. Drain over a bowl and press the water from the hijiki with the back of a large spoon. Heat 1 tablespoon of the oil in a medium skillet over high heat and sauté the hijiki for 2 minutes. Add all but the last inch of the reserved soaking liquid, plus water to cover. Simmer until tender, about 1 minute. Drain and set aside.

Pick through the crab to remove any shell fragments. In a small skillet, heat 1 tablespoon of the oil over high heat and sauté the red pepper until limp. Set aside to cool.

In a blender or food processor, process the bread into crumbs. In a medium bowl, combine the crabmeat, hijiki, peppers, garlic, jalapeño, cilantro, and cabbage leaf. Add the filé or seasoning, 2 tablespoons of the bread crumbs, salt, and pepper.

Mix well, cover, and refrigerate for 20 minutes.

Sprinkle the remaining bread crumbs on waxed paper. Using an ice cream scoop or large spoon, form 8 equal portions of crab mixture. Pat each into a ¾-inch-thick disk. Press each cake into the bread crumbs, coating evenly on both sides. Refrigerate for 1 hour.

Preheat the oven to 375°F. Heat a large cast-iron skillet in the oven for 30 minutes. Add the remaining oil to the pan and heat over high heat until it smokes. Place the crab cakes gently in the pan, leaving space between them, and cook until well browned on each side. Transfer the pan to the oven and bake the cakes for 6 minutes.

To make the sauce: Combine the mayonnaise and horseradish and serve alongside the crab cakes.

Skewered Chicken
WITH HOT PEANUT SAUCE

Makes 8 appetizer servings or 4 main-dish servings

This variation on a classic Southeast Asian dish was created by Linda Hillel. Serve as an appetizer or as a main course with fragrant jasmine or basmati rice.

½ cup unsalted chunky peanut butter

1 tablespoon Asian sesame oil

1½ teaspoons chili oil, or more to taste

3 tablespoons mirin (sweet sake) or dry sherry

2 tablespoons low-salt soy sauce

2 tablespoons grated fresh ginger

1½ pounds skinless, boneless chicken breasts, cut into 1-inch strips

2 tablespoons plain rice vinegar

3 tablespoons minced fresh cilantro

In a small bowl, combine the peanut butter, oils, mirin or sherry, soy sauce, and ginger; stir to blend. In a large bowl, toss the chicken with about one third of the peanut sauce mixture and reserve the rest. Cover and refrigerate for at least 1 hour or up to 6 hours. Stir the vinegar and cilantro into the reserved peanut sauce and set aside.

Remove the chicken from the refrigerator 30 minutes before grilling. Light a fire in a charcoal or gas grill. Thread the chicken strips lengthwise on skewers. Grill the chicken over hot coals for 1 or 2 minutes on each side, or until opaque throughout.

Serve with reserved peanut sauce on the side.

CHILI FENNEL SPRING ROLLS

Makes 8 servings

Both hot and cool, these tasty rolls are nearly transparent, brimming with light, springy garden greens. This is a terrific way to serve fennel, which is rich in phytoestrogens.

1 cup sliced cooked chicken or beef

2 teaspoons plain rice vinegar

¼ teaspoon chili oil

1 tablespoon fresh lime juice

8 rice paper sheets

½ cup fennel bulb, trimmed

½ cup chopped fresh cilantro

½ cup chopped green onion, including the green parts

½ cup shredded outer leaves of Chinese cabbage

Soy sauce for serving

Place the cooked chicken or beef in a mixing bowl with the rice vinegar, chili oil, and lime juice. Turn several times until coated.

Soak the rice paper in a bowl of cool water to cover until pliable, about 5 minutes. Gently remove the sheets and drain on paper towels.

With a thin, sharp knife, cut the fennel bulb along the grain until a thin "ribbon" of fennel curls up. Combine the cilantro, green onion, and cabbage.

Place on a serving platter. Fill each sheet with 1 heaping tablespoon greens and 1 heaping tablespoon meat. Roll up each sheet, pinching the bottom to keep it together. Serve with soy sauce.

Black Bean and Tofu Wraps

Makes 36 appetizers

Glistening black beans lend deep color, texture, and unique taste to this lively salsa, which is delicious with lightly warmed tortillas.

6 small flour tortillas

1 cup Black Bean and Tofu Relish (see page 69)

Place the tortillas directly on the oven racks of a preheated 425°F oven. Lay the warmed tortillas on a work surface. Spread 3 tablespoons of the bean mixture on each tortilla. Roll into a tight tube. Using a very sharp knife, slice the rolls into 1-inch lengths and arrange on a platter.

LEEK WRAPS

Makes 14 to 16 appetizers

2 large leeks, white part only

2 tablespoons olive oil

1 tablespoon black mustard seed

1 onion, finely chopped

¼ teaspoon ground coriander

1 teaspoon fresh lemon juice

3 tablespoons capers, drained

3 large flour tortillas

¼ cup chopped fresh parsley

In a covered steamer or saucepan, steam the leeks over boiling water until tender, about 5 minutes. Let cool and dice.

In a medium skillet, heat the oil over high heat. Add the mustard seed and cook until popped, but not burned. Add the onion and cook until tender, about 2 minutes. Stir in the coriander, lemon juice, capers, and leeks. Cook for 3 minutes, stirring to blend.

Warm tortillas for 2 minutes in a 425°F oven. Keep covered with a damp cloth until ready to use.

Lay the tortillas flat on a work surface. Spread one third of the leek mixture on each tortilla and roll tightly into a tube. Cut crosswise into 1-inch lengths. Arrange on a platter and garnish with parsley.

CELERY LEAF AND OLIVE CROSTINI

Makes 6 servings

Calcium-rich cottage cheese is the topping for this appetizer by Linda Hillel. Rich olives and crunchy celery add taste contrast.

1 garlic clove, pressed

3 tablespoons extra-virgin olive oil

1 long sourdough loaf or baguette,
    cut into ½-inch-thick diagonal slices

1 cup low-fat cottage cheese

¼ cup oil-packed or oil-cured black olives, pitted

1 cup celery leaves

½ teaspoon pepper

½ teaspoon dried rosemary or marjoram

Preheat the oven to 400°F. Combine the garlic and oil in a small bowl. Brush onto one side of the bread slices and bake on a baking sheet until lightly browned, about 10 minutes.

Meanwhile, put the remaining ingredients in a blender or food processor and pulse to chop and combine. Transfer to an ovenproof dish and place in the oven for 1 to 2 minutes to warm slightly. Spread on the bread slices and serve immediately.

GREEN TOFU BRUSCHETTA

Makes 6 servings

Steamed spicy greens, tofu, sesame oil, and garlic blend in this
fresh mustard green pesto by Linda Hillel. Healthful yet hearty,
it is perfect for parties.

**4 ounces mustard or dandelion greens,
 stemmed and finely chopped**

1 baguette or ½ loaf French bread, sliced ½ inch thick

2 unpeeled garlic cloves, halved diagonally

8 ounces soft tofu, rinsed and drained

1½ tablespoons Asian sesame oil

2 tablespoons fresh lemon juice

1 tablespoon Dijon mustard

Kosher salt and freshly ground pepper to taste

Dash of chili oil or cayenne pepper to taste (optional)

Preheat the oven to 350°F. In a covered steamer or saucepan, steam the
greens over boiling water until tender, about 5 minutes. Drain, squeeze out the
excess liquid, and set aside.

Place the bread slices on a baking sheet and bake until lightly browned,
about 4 minutes. Rub one side of each slice with garlic and set aside.

In a small bowl, thoroughly combine the cooked greens with all the remaining ingredients. Spread on the garlic-rubbed side of each bruschetta.

Variation: Press ½ garlic clove, add to the tofu mixture, and serve as a dip
with toasted pita wedges.

Smoky Tofu Pizza

Makes 6 to 8 appetizer servings or 2 main-course servings

Tofu and vegetables, lightly sprinkled with smoked cheese for flavor, top this pizza by Linda Hillel. Serve as an appetizer, sliced into thin wedges, or as a main course, with salad.

2 tablespoons olive oil

1 onion, thinly sliced

2 garlic cloves, pressed

10 ounces portobello or
    other fresh mushrooms, sliced

1 *each* red and yellow bell pepper, seeded,
    deribbed, and cut into julienne strips

1 teaspoon dried rosemary, crumbled

¼ teaspoon dried oregano
    or marjoram

¼ teaspoon dried thyme

7 ounces firm tofu, rinsed, drained,
    and mashed with a fork

Kosher salt and freshly ground
    pepper to taste

1 large pizza crust or focaccia,
    or several smaller ones

1 cup (4 ounces) freshly grated
    smoked cheese such as smoked mozzarella

reheat the oven to 400°F.

Heat the oil in a large sauté pan or skillet over medium-high heat. Add the onion, garlic, mushrooms, peppers, and herbs. Sauté until the vegetables are tender, about 5 to 7 minutes.

Add the tofu, salt, and pepper. Spread evenly on each crust or focaccia. Sprinkle with grated cheese. Bake on a pizza pan or baking sheet for 8 to 10 minutes, or until the cheese melts. If desired, place under the broiler for 1 or 2 minutes, or until browned.

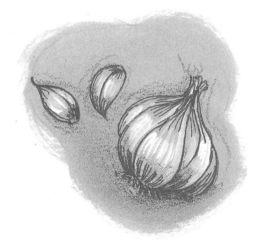

Appetizers

FENNEL CAPONATA PIZZA

Makes 16 appetizers

This quick, Mediterranean appetizer makes a great light lunch
with a little goat cheese crumbled on top and a salad on the side.

2 prebaked packaged 6-inch pizza crusts

1 teaspoon olive oil

¼ cup diced fennel stalk

1 cup bottled caponata

2 tablespoons pine nuts

Minced fresh chives for garnish

Preheat the oven to 500°F. Place the crusts on a baking sheet large enough
for both and bake for 3 to 5 minutes.

Heat the oil in a small skillet over medium-high heat and sauté the fennel
for 2 minutes, or until tender. Drain.

Spread the crusts with caponata. Scatter with pine nuts and fennel and bake
for 2 minutes, or until the nuts turn golden. Garnish with chives and cut each
pizza into 8 slices. Serve at once.

SOUPS

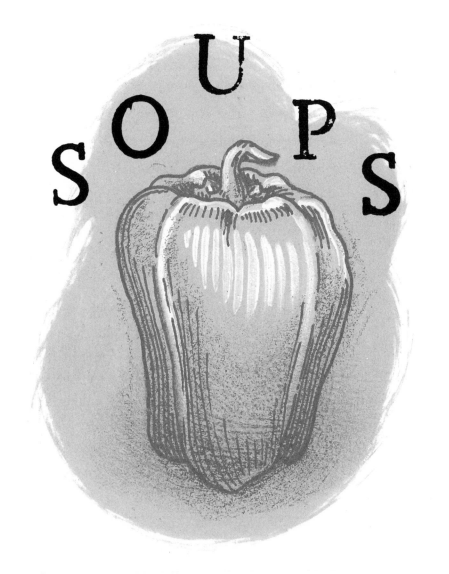

CHILLED LEMON-MISO SOUP

Makes 4 servings

The pale lemon shade of this soup looks delicate but harbors a robust array of nutrients.

1 carrot, peeled and cut into thin slices

6½ cups nonfat chicken broth

½ cup chicken bones

2½ tablespoons white miso paste

3 tablespoons fresh lemon juice

3 tablespoons white wine vinegar

3 scallions, including the green part,
   finely chopped

Minced carrot leaves for garnish

10 ounces tofu, cut into small cubes,
   for garnish (optional)

In a covered steamer or saucepan, cook the carrot over boiling water until tender, about 3 minutes. In a large pot, bring the broth and bones to a boil. Remove 1 cup of the liquid and add the miso to the pot, stirring to dissolve. Strain the broth to remove the bones. Add the lemon juice, vinegar, cooked carrot, and scallions. Cover and refrigerate for 1 or 2 hours, or until chilled. Serve garnished with carrot leaves and tofu, if desired.

CREAMY ASPARAGUS SOUP WITH FENNEL

Makes 6 first-course servings or 3 main-course servings

Thickened with grains, this elegant and robustly flavored soup by Linda Hillel uses all parts of the fennel plant. Asparagus was prized by the Greeks and Romans for its unique flavor.

1 fennel bulb

1 pound asparagus, trimmed

1 tablespoon vegetable oil

1 onion, sliced

½ cup brown rice or pearl barley

4 cups nonfat chicken broth or low-salt vegetable broth

1½ cups low-fat milk

Salt and freshly ground pepper to taste

Separate the fennel fronds from the bulb and stems. Finely mince the fronds to make ½ cup. Slice the fennel bulb and stems.

Cut off 1½ inches of the asparagus tips. Peel the asparagus stalks with a vegetable peeler, then cut into 1-inch pieces.

In a large saucepan over medium-high heat, heat the oil and sauté the sliced fennel stems, asparagus stalks, and onion for 5 minutes. Add the rice or barley and broth, cover, and cook over low heat 30 to 40 minutes, or until the rice or barley is very tender.

Transfer to a blender or food processor and puree to the desired consistency in several batches if necessary. Return the puree to the pan and stir in 1 cup of the milk, the reserved fennel fronds, the asparagus tips, salt, and pepper. If the soup seems too thick, stir in a little more of the milk. Heat until the asparagus tips are crisp-tender, about 1½ minutes.

CREAMY CARROT
AND WHITE BEAN SOUP

Makes 4 servings

In this recipe, beans bring a rich store of potassium to prompt surges of extra energy, while tofu teems with soy phytoestrogens. The combination of beans, tofu, and carrots is delicious.

1 teaspoon olive oil

1 small onion, finely chopped

2 garlic cloves, minced

1 cup dried Great Northern beans,
   soaked overnight and drained

7 cups water

1 large fresh rosemary sprig

2 large fresh thyme sprigs

1½ cups diced peeled carrots

10 roasted garlic cloves (see Note)

10 ounces soft or firm tofu,
   rinsed and drained

1¼ teaspoons salt, or to taste

Freshly ground pepper to taste

¼ teaspoon cayenne pepper

GARNISH 1 teaspoon rosemary olive oil or
extra-virgin olive oil

½ teaspoon grated lemon zest

4 small fresh rosemary sprigs

eat the oil in a large saucepan over medium heat. Add the onion and cook until tender, about 5 minutes. Add the garlic and, stirring constantly, cook for 30 seconds. Add the beans and water and bring to a boil. Add the rosemary and thyme, cover, and simmer for 40 minutes.

Stir in the carrots and roasted garlic. Cook for 25 more minutes, or until the beans are tender. Drain the beans, reserving the liquid. Put the beans, tofu, and 3 cups of the reserved liquid in a blender or food processor and puree until smooth. Add more liquid if desired. Save any leftover liquid for soup stock.

Return the puree to the saucepan and simmer, stirring constantly, for 5 minutes. Do not allow it to boil. Add the salt, pepper, and cayenne. Ladle the soup into 4 bowls. Drizzle ¼ teaspoon rosemary oil and a little lemon zest over each. Garnish with rosemary.

Note: To roast garlic, put separated cloves on a baking sheet and drizzle with oilive oil. Roast in a 450°F oven for 6 to 10 minutes, depending on size of cloves. Cool and peel.

Iced Dill-Cucumber Soup

Makes 6 servings

The light green hue of this soup reflects its cool and refreshing flavor, making it the perfect choice for hot summer weather. Sorrel lends an unusual lemony piquancy.

2½ cups water

1 cup low-salt vegetable broth
  or nonfat chicken broth

6 cucumbers, peeled and cut into 1½-inch slices

2 teaspoons minced fresh dill weed

1 tablespoon minced sorrel

2 tablespoons grated lemon zest

1 tablespoon minced lemon membrane
  and pulp

1 tablespoon white miso paste

Juice of 1 lemon

6 fresh fennel fronds

6 fresh lemon slices

In a large saucepan, bring the water and broth to a boil. Lower heat and add the cucumbers, dill, sorrel, lemon zest, membrane, and pulp; simmer until tender. Transfer to a blender or food processor and puree with the miso and lemon juice, adding more water if a thinner soup is desired. Cover and refrigerate for 2 hours or more. Garnish with fennel fronds and lemon slices.

GINGER-TOFU SOUP

Makes 4 large servings

Bright, spicy flavor combines with chile, chicken, tamarind juice, and fish sauce in this exotic soup. Fish sauce *(nam pla)* and tamarind juice are available in Asian markets.

½ tablespoon minced garlic

½ jalapeño chile, minced

¼ cup cilantro roots, minced

1 pound firm tofu, rinsed, drained, and cut into ½-inch cubes

3 cups nonfat chicken broth

¼ cup fish sauce

¼ cup chopped onion

6 tablespoons tamarind juice

¼ cup sliced and peeled fresh ginger

4 tablespoons sugar

½ cup chopped green onions, including the green part

Fresh cilantro leaves for garnish

With a mortar and pestle, mash the garlic, jalapeño, and cilantro roots to a thick paste.

In a large stockpot, heat the chicken broth to a simmer and add all the ingredients except the green onions and cilantro leaves. Cook for 10 minutes. Remove from heat, add the green onions, and garnish with cilantro leaves.

SOY BROTH
WITH BITTER GREENS AND GINGER

Makes 4 servings

Cool longevity is a midlife motto, which applies to ginger as well. Keep ginger cool to preserve its immune-boosting and cardiovascular-enhancing properties.

4 cups nonfat chicken broth

¼ cup dry sherry or vermouth

¼ cup low-salt soy sauce

2 tablespoons chopped and peeled fresh ginger

2 lemongrass stalks

¼ teaspoon red pepper flakes

¼ cup chopped dandelion leaves

½ cup sugar snap peas

In a large saucepan, heat the chicken broth to boiling. Add the sherry or vermouth, soy, ginger, lemongrass, and pepper flakes. Boil for 1 more minute. Remove from heat and add the dandelions and snap peas. Cover and let sit for 3 minutes. Remove the lemongrass before serving.

ORANGE-FENNEL REFRESCO

Makes about 4 cups

Serene as a sea breeze, this cool compote has a refreshing color
and taste. The tart citrus and mellow fennel mixture can be
spooned over vegetables or served with rice as a condiment.

1 cup fresh orange juice

½ teaspoon minced orange membrane
   and pulp (see page 45)

1 cup dry white wine

2 tablespoons balsamic vinegar

3 fresh basil leaves

6 shallots, coarsely chopped

½ cup slivered fennel stems

4 navel oranges, peeled and thinly sliced

Place all the ingredients except the oranges in a blender or food processor
and blend rapidly for 20 seconds. Stir the mixture briefly, scraping down the
sides, then blend again for another 20 seconds. The mixture should be somewhat coarse, not a smooth puree. Transfer to a covered container and set aside.

Place the orange slices in the blender or food processor and blend rapidly
for 30 seconds. Stir, then blend again for 30 seconds. Add to the compote and
combine thoroughly. Refrigerate for 2 to 4 hours before serving.

Green Apple and Almond Soup

Makes 4 servings

Good warm or cold, this singular soup has a warm and spicy holiday fragrance as well as a festive minty color. Almonds add delicious texture and nutty appeal.

5 Granny Smith or Pippin apples, peeled, cored, and chopped (reserve peels and cores)

3 cups apple juice

2 cinnamon sticks

2½ cups water

2 tablespoons butter

1¼ cups (6 ounces) chopped blanched almonds

2 large garlic cloves, crushed

1½ cups chopped onions

½ teaspoon minced fresh ginger

1 teaspoon salt

Juice of 1 lemon

3 tablespoons flour

1 teaspoon dry mustard

1 teaspoon ground turmeric

1 teaspoon ground cumin

1 teaspoon fennel seed

½ teaspoon ground coriander

¼ teaspoon ground cloves

Freshly ground pepper to taste

2 cups plain nonfat yogurt

1 pound soft tofu, rinsed and drained

In a large pot, combine the apple peels and cores, apple juice, cinnamon sticks, and water. Bring to a boil, then simmer, partially covered, for 45 minutes. Remove from heat and let stand for 1 hour. Strain and reserve the liquid.

In a heavy skillet, melt the butter over low heat and sauté the almonds, garlic, and onions until the almonds are toasted, about 8 to 10 minutes. Remove the almond mixture from the skillet and set aside. Add the apples, ginger, salt, and lemon juice to the skillet and cook for 3 minutes over medium-high heat. Add the flour and spices and stir to combine thoroughly. Cover and cook an additional 8 to 10 minutes over low heat. Remove from heat and let rest about 10 minutes. While the fruit mixture is resting, reheat the apple juice liquid over medium heat.

In a blender, puree the almonds with a little of the liquid. When thoroughly blended, add the apples and the rest of the liquid, blending until smooth. If thinner soup is preferred, a little more water may be added. Transfer the soup to a heavy saucepan. Combine the yogurt and tofu, then whisk into the mixture without further cooking. Keep warm over low heat until ready to serve.

Mango-Avocado Gazpacho

Makes 4 to 6 servings

Avocado and mango combine beautifully in this delicious summer soup. The unusual light green color and velvety texture are soothing and cool, and the soup is loaded with vitamin E.

2 cucumbers,
  cut into ½-inch-thick slices

1 large ripe mango, peeled, pitted,
  and cut into ½-inch-thick slices

4 whole scallions, minced

1 garlic clove, crushed

½ cup minced fresh parsley

1 tablespoon minced fresh cilantro

1 large ripe avocado

Juice of 2 limes
  (about 6 tablespoons)

1 cup cold water

1 tablespoon salt

Freshly ground pepper to taste

1 tablespoon minced fresh basil

2 tablespoons olive oil

1 tablespoon sugar

Combine the cucumbers, mango slices, and scallions in a large bowl. Add the garlic, parsley, and cilantro.

In a separate bowl, mash the avocado with the lime juice. Add to the mango mixture and combine thoroughly. Place one third of this mixture in a blender or food processor and puree until smooth. Stir the puree into the mango mixture. Cover and refrigerate for at least 1 hour. Serve cold.

Smoky Yam and Cilantro Soup

Makes 4 servings

This soup begins its life on the barbecue. The smoky essence of fire and lime suggest banked embers on a starlit night.

2 yams, peeled and
   cut into quarters

½ cup wood chips

1 cup milk

1½ cups nonfat chicken broth

Juice of 1 lime

⅛ teaspoon red pepper flakes

Dash *each* of ground nutmeg,
   cumin, and pepper

Salt to taste

3 tablespoons Madeira wine
   (optional)

½ bunch fresh cilantro,
   stemmed and chopped

Grated lime zest for garnish

In a covered steamer or saucepan, steam the yams over boiling water for about 6 minutes, or until barely tender. Let cool.

Soak the wood chips in water to cover for at least 30 minutes. Prepare a fire in a charcoal grill. When the coals are white-hot, drain the wood chips and sprinkle them over the coals. Place the yams on the grill and cook for 10 minutes, turning twice. Cook longer for a stronger, smokier flavor. The yams will darken and mottle, but this only enhances the soup's appearance.

In a blender or food processor, puree the yams. Add the milk and 1 cup of the chicken broth and puree. Pour into a large saucepan and simmer over low heat to thicken. Add the lime juice, red pepper flakes, nutmeg, cumin, pepper, and salt. Add the Madeira, if desired. The soup should have a glistening, thick surface. If too thick, add the remaining ½ cup broth. Garnish with cilantro and lime zest.

Soups

MOROCCAN CHICKEN SOUP

Makes 4 to 6 servings

Tasty, traditional, and steeped with rich nutrients, this soup by
Lalia Mohamed is a filling dinner or, served in small bowls, a
savory appetizer with pita wedges.

1 tablespoon virgin olive oil

1 large onion, chopped

1 small chicken, cut up, skin and fat removed

2 tablespoons ground caraway seeds

½ teaspoon ground cinnamon

1 tablespoon pepper

2½ teaspoons salt

2 small zucchini, cut into ¼-inch-thick slices

2 carrots, peeled and cut into ¼-inch-thick slices

2 potatoes, cut crosswise into ½-inch-thick slices

1 bunch fresh cilantro, stemmed and chopped

5 tablespoons tomato paste

6 cups water

½ cup fresh peas

½ cup fresh lemon juice

Lemon wedges for garnish

In a large, heavy pot, heat the oil over medium heat and sauté the onion and chicken for 2 minutes, or until browned. Lower heat and add the caraway seeds, cinnamon, pepper, and salt. Mix well and sauté for 2 to 3 more minutes. Add all the remaining ingredients except the peas, lemon juice, and lemon wedges. Cover and bring to a boil. Lower heat and simmer gently until the chicken is tender, about 30 minutes. Transfer the chicken pieces to a plate and let cool to the touch. Set aside.

Puree the soup in a blender or food processor, then return to the pot. Bring to a boil, add the peas, and cook for 3 minutes. Meanwhile, remove the chicken meat from the bones and return it to the soup. Add the lemon juice to the soup, stir to combine, and serve with lemon wedges.

Yam Silk Soup

Makes 4 servings

Luscious and thick, this rich golden soup is a harvest offering of sweet corn, yam, and squash, with a genial dash of added spice.

1 onion, thinly sliced

4 shallots, sliced

¼ teaspoon salt

2 garlic cloves, minced

1 pound butternut squash, peeled, seeded, and cubed (3 cups)

1 yam (3 to 6 ounces), peeled and cubed

1 cup fresh corn kernels (about 2 ears)

½ cup chicken broth

1 teaspoon olive oil

1 teaspoon dried thyme

Dash *each* of ground ginger and allspice

Freshly ground white pepper to taste

GARNISH Shaved fresh ginger

Julienned red bell pepper

n a large sauté pan or skillet over medium-high heat, heat the olive oil and sauté the onion, shallots, and salt until the onion is translucent, about 5 minutes. Add the garlic and cook for 2 minutes. Stir in the squash, yam, corn, and thyme. Add water to cover. Bring to a boil, then lower heat and cook, uncovered, for 3 minutes. Transfer to a blender or food processor, add the broth, and puree until smooth. Season with the spices and garnish with the ginger and red pepper.

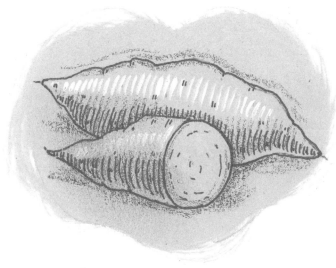

Soups

SAL ADS

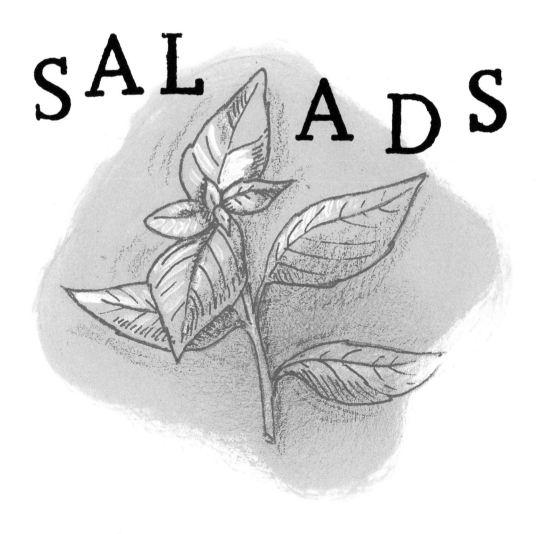

CHIPOTLE-ORANGE SALAD

Makes 6 servings

Chipotle chiles add a smoky Southwestern touch to orange slices layered with red onion, Belgian endive, goat cheese, and arugula. The flavors are dark yet strong, making the salad an ideal accompaniment to lamb or pork.

2 bunches arugula

1 small head Belgian endive,
   thinly sliced

3 thin slices red onion,
   separated into rings

3 ounces fresh white goat cheese,
   crumbled

2 tablespoons flaxseed

1 tablespoon sesame seeds,
   toasted (see page 55)

1 tablespoon sunflower seeds,
   toasted (see page 55)

ORANGE
DRESSING

¼ teaspoon grated orange zest

½ cup fresh orange juice

⅛ teaspoon minced orange pulp
   and membrane (see page 45)

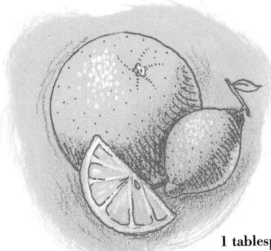

1 tablespoon champagne vinegar

2 tablespoons extra-virgin olive oil

2 tablespoons Dijon mustard

1 teaspoon minced canned chipotle chile en adobo

⅛ teaspoon salt

In a large salad bowl, combine the arugula and endive. Add the onion rings, cheese, and seeds. Toss gently.

To make the dressing: Combine all the ingredients in a small bowl. Drizzle a little dressing over the salad and serve the rest on the side.

Sicilian Orange-Pepper Plate

Makes 4 servings

Sunny oranges sprinkled with pepper flakes and marinated in red wine make a hearty, rustic dish. Serve as a side salad or a healthful dessert.

4 plump blood oranges

1 garlic clove, halved

2 tablespoons corn oil

3 to 4 tablespoons dry red wine

½ teaspoon balsamic or red wine vinegar

¼ teaspoon red pepper flakes

Salt and freshly ground pepper to taste

2 tablespoons pine nuts, toasted (see page 52)

Score the oranges with a sharp knife and peel, section, and seed them. Carefully remove the white inner membrane from the peeled oranges. Mince the membrane to make ½ teaspoon; set aside.

Rub the inside of a bowl with 1 garlic half. Cut the orange segments with a sharp knife, then place in the bowl and stir in the minced membrane and all the remaining ingredients except the nuts. Let sit for 5 to 10 minutes. Sprinkle with nuts before serving.

Moroccan Orange-Walnut Salad

Makes 2 to 4 servings

Leafy green spinach, olive oil, and walnuts are all rich in vitamin E, while potassium-rich oranges give an energy spike. The orange flower water adds an aromatic touch to this dish, which is perfect for a lunch.

6 large navel oranges

1 tablespoon honey

½ teaspoon ground cinnamon

½ teaspoon orange flower water (optional)

1 pound mixed fresh spinach, romaine, and arugula leaves

½ cup thinly sliced red onion

1 cup thinly sliced radishes

1 cup walnut halves, toasted (see pages 52–53)

3 tablespoons extra-virgin olive oil

Salt and freshly ground pepper to taste

Peel, section, and seed the oranges, reserving the pulp and membrane. Mince ½ tablespoon of the membrane and set aside. Drizzle the honey and cinnamon over the oranges, then add the orange flower water, if desired. Cover and let sit at room temperature for 1 hour.

Combine the greens in a large bowl with the onion, radishes, and nuts. Sprinkle with olive oil and toss. Season with salt and pepper.

Pear-Daikon Salad

Makes 4 servings

Daikon radish adds a spicy kick to this exuberant dish. A sprinkle of lemon juice preserves the light, clear color of the pears in this make-ahead salad.

1 bunch arugula (10 to 12 ounces)

One 3-inch piece daikon (Japanese white radish), peeled

½ very ripe pear, peeled, cored, and cut into chunks

1 teaspoon fresh lemon juice

1 tablespoon safflower oil

Pinch of ground cumin

Kosher salt and freshly ground pepper to taste

Tear the arugula into pieces and place in a salad bowl. Using a vegetable peeler, shave the daikon into long ribbons. Toss with the arugula.

Push the pear through a sieve with the back of a wooden spoon into a small bowl to make a thick puree. Stir in the lemon juice, oil, and cumin. Add the salt and pepper. Add to the arugula mixture, toss, and serve.

Cool Fennel Salad

Makes 8 servings

A quick salad that offers the unexpected contrast of salty cheese and cool licorice taste.

2 tablespoons fresh lemon juice

¼ teaspoon pepper

¼ cup olive oil

2 fennel bulbs, trimmed

½ cup (2 ounces) grated Parmesan cheese

In a small bowl, combine the lemon juice and pepper. Whisk in the olive oil until thoroughly blended and set aside.

Slice the fennel bulbs lengthwise into thin strips and arrange them on salad plates. Drizzle the fennel strips with the vinaigrette and sprinkle with Parmesan.

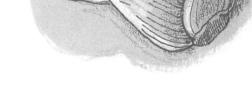

Mood Swing Antipasto

Serves 2 to 4

Onion and fennel complement one another in a delicious harmony, studded with peppercorns for spicy contrast.

¼ **cup plain rice vinegar**

¼ **cup water**

½ **bay leaf**

10 whole black peppercorns

1 small red onion, thinly sliced

1 fennel bulb, trimmed and thinly sliced

**1 bunch arugula (10 to 12 ounces),
stemmed and shredded**

In a small saucepan, combine the vinegar, water, bay leaf, and peppercorns. Bring to a boil and cook for 10 minutes.

Place the onion and fennel slices in separate bowls and pour half the vinegar mixture over each. Let sit for 1 hour at room temperature. Cover and refrigerate until ready to serve. Serve mounded separately on a bed of arugula.

Blood Orange, Fennel,
AND GOAT CHEESE SALAD

Makes 4 servings

A cool and composed salad for the cool and composed midlife woman. This fennel dish by Linda Hillel blends mellow fennel with robust cheese and pepper for contrast.

2 blood oranges

3 tablespoons extra-virgin olive oil

1 teaspoon honey

Salt and freshly ground pepper
  to taste

1 fennel bulb with fronds

½ cup fresh white goat cheese
  (plain or with herbs or pepper),
  crumbled

¼ cup walnuts, toasted and coarsely
  chopped (see pages 52–53)

Halve 1 orange and juice one half. Cut off the peel of the remaining 1½ oranges down to the flesh with a knife. Cut the oranges into thin slices and set aside.

In a medium bowl, whisk together the orange juice, oil, honey, salt, and pepper. Mince about 1 tablespoon of the fennel fronds and stir into the dressing.

Trim the fennel bulb and cut it into paper-thin slices. (Save the stems and remaining fronds for another use.)

Toss the fennel with the dressing. With a slotted spoon, divide the fennel among 4 salad plates. Arrange the orange slices around or on the fennel. Top with the goat cheese. Spoon some of the dressing from the bowl evenly over each salad. Sprinkle with the nuts.

KALE AND ARUGULA SALAD
WITH GOAT CHEESE

Makes 4 servings

Lemony, tart, invigorating, and hearty, this salad is a complete meal in itself.

4 ounces fresh white goat cheese

3 slices bacon or Canadian bacon, diced

1 bunch kale, trimmed and cut into strips

1 garlic clove, minced

¼ cup plain rice vinegar

1 tablespoon champagne vinegar

3 tablespoons Asian sesame oil

Pinch of grated lemon zest and minced lemon membrane (see page 45)

⅛ teaspoon cumin seeds, crushed

Dash of ground cinnamon

Warmed pita bread, cut into wedges, for serving

Preheat the oven to 300°F for 10 minutes. Turn off the oven. Place the goat cheese in a covered casserole or cover with foil and place on a baking pan. Place in the oven to warm.

In a small skillet, sauté the bacon pieces over high heat until crisp. Using a slotted spoon, transfer to paper towels to drain. Pour the fat out of the pan and return the bacon to the pan. Add the garlic, cook briefly, then add the kale and cook until limp. Transfer to a salad bowl.

In a small bowl, mix the vinegars, oil, lemon zest and membrane, and spices. Drizzle over the warm kale and toss. To serve, cut the warm goat cheese in fourths and place one piece on top of each salad. Serve with pita bread.

Cucumber, Green Bean,
and Wakame Salad

Makes 4 to 5 servings

Peaceful as a garden, this calming combination highlights savory greens. An unusual medley of crisp beans and cucumbers scattered with deep green wakame, this savory mingling of flavors is rich in vitamin E.

3 cucumbers, peeled and
   cut into ¼-inch-thick slices

8 ounces green beans,
   steamed and cooled

½ teaspoon salt

4 ounces wakame, chopped (½ cup)

½ cup water

6 tablespoons plain rice vinegar

2 tablespoons mirin (sweet sake)
   or dry sherry

2 tablespoons olive oil

¼ teaspoon ground ginger

¼ cup chopped fresh chives

⅛ cup thinly sliced
   preserved red radishes
   (available in Asian markets)

1 teaspoon minced garlic

¼ teaspoon green peppercorns

8 ounces mixed baby greens

Sunflower seeds, toasted,
   for garnish (see page 55)

Place the cucumber slices in a large bowl. Cut the green beans lengthwise into thin slices and add to the cucumbers. Add all the remaining ingredients except the greens and sunflower seeds. Cover and refrigerate overnight.

Serve on a bed of greens and garnish with sunflower seeds.

ENDIVE, FIG, AND GOAT CHEESE SALAD
WITH POMEGRANATE VINAIGRETTE

Makes 4 servings

Japanese women on tofu-rich diets seldom experience hot flashes. What better way to enjoy this vital food than with the crunch of endive and the sweet succulence of figs? This luxurious dish is heartily scattered with walnuts and brightened with a vivid red vinaigrette.

VINAIGRETTE

1 pomegranate, halved

½ cup plain rice vinegar

2 tablespoons fresh lemon juice

½ cup walnuts, chopped

3 tablespoons water

Salt and freshly ground black pepper to taste

8 fresh figs

1 head curly endive, cut into bite-sized pieces

4 ounces soft tofu, rinsed and drained

8 ounces fresh white goat cheese at room temperature

½ cup fresh bread crumbs

To make the vinaigrette: Squeeze the juice from each pomegranate half using a lemon juicer. Add the rice vinegar and lemon juice. Whisk or shake until thoroughly blended.

Preheat the oven to 350°F. Spread the walnuts on a baking sheet, sprinkle lightly with the water, and lightly season with salt and pepper. Bake until toasty brown, about 7 minutes. Cut the figs in quarters but leave them attached at the base. Arrange the figs and endive on salad plates and drizzle with the vinaigrette.

Blend the tofu and goat cheese, using a spoon or a pastry cutter. Form into 4 patties and coat with the bread crumbs. Place 1 patty on each bed of endive and sprinkle with the walnuts.

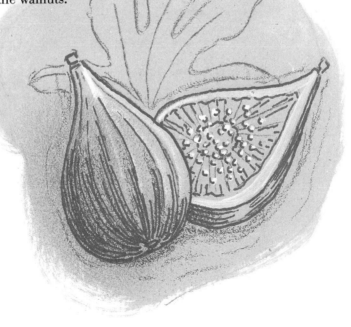

Salads

Fish Salad with Peanut-Tofu Dressing

Makes 4 servings

Peanut sauce is a joyous flavor splash for mild-tasting fish and tofu in this contemporary salad by Linda Hillel. An artful mixture of cold fish, brisk arugula, and scattered peanuts.

PEANUT-
TOFU
DRESSING

1 small garlic clove, pressed

2 tablespoons minced fresh ginger

2 tablespoons unsalted peanut butter

1 tablespoon low-salt soy sauce

2 tablespoons mirin (sweet sake) or dry sherry

2 tablespoons plain rice vinegar

½ teaspoon chili oil, or to taste

2 teaspoons Asian sesame oil

⅓ cup chopped fresh cilantro

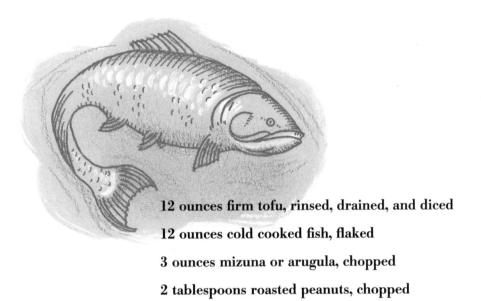

12 ounces firm tofu, rinsed, drained, and diced

12 ounces cold cooked fish, flaked

3 ounces mizuna or arugula, chopped

2 tablespoons roasted peanuts, chopped

To make the dressing: Combine all the ingredients in a blender or food processor and blend until smooth.

In a large bowl, gently combine the tofu, fish, and greens. Drizzle with the peanut dressing and toss lightly. Garnish with the chopped peanuts.

Smoked Chicken
and Pepita Salad

Makes 6 servings

The delicate flavor of toasted pumpkin seeds belies their intensely rich component of vitamin E. Choose organic chicken for its superior flavor and purer nutrition.

MARINADE   ⅔ cup olive oil

½ cup fresh lime juice

1 jalapeño chile, seeded and minced

¼ cup dry white wine

6 skinless, boneless chicken breast halves

½ cup mesquite wood chips

PEPITAS   1 cup unsalted green pumpkin seeds

2 tablespoons fresh lime juice

¼ teaspoon ground cumin

Salt and freshly ground pepper to taste

DRESSING   ⅓ cup olive oil

1 garlic clove, minced

2 green onions, including the green part,
   finely chopped

1 tablespoon fresh lemon juice

1 tablespoon fresh lime juice

1 tablespoon orange juice

½ teaspoon red pepper flakes

GARNISH   2 bunches arugula

Mix the marinade ingredients together in a shallow nonaluminum pan. Add the chicken and coat with marinade. Cover and refrigerate for 4 hours, turning the chicken several times.

Soak the mesquite in water to cover for 30 minutes. Remove the chicken from the refrigerator 30 minutes before cooking. Light a fire in a charcoal grill. When the coals are hot, drain the chips and sprinkle them over the coals. Grill the chicken in the covered grill for about 4 minutes on each side, or until opaque throughout.

To make the pepitas: Preheat the oven to 200°F. Spread the seeds on a baking sheet and toast until crisp, about 15 minutes. In a small bowl, toss the toasted seeds with the lime, cumin, salt, and pepper and set aside.

In a small bowl, whisk the dressing ingredients together. Refrigerate if not using immediately.

Cut the chicken into strips and place on a bed of arugula. Drizzle with dressing and scatter with pumpkin seeds.

CHINESE CABBAGE SALAD

Makes 4 to 6 servings

A day's rest before serving allows the sweet and sour flavors of this salad to meld and mingle. Green onions and potassium-rich peanuts are a crisp final addition.

½ cup smooth natural peanut butter

½ cup hot water

½ cup plus 1 tablespoon plain rice vinegar

3 tablespoons packed brown sugar

½ teaspoon salt

1 tablespoon low-salt soy sauce

1 teaspoon Asian sesame oil

7 to 8 cups green cabbage,
   including the outer leaves, shredded

Cayenne pepper to taste

4 ounces unsalted roasted peanuts, crushed

3 green onions, including the green part, chopped

In a large bowl, mix the peanut butter and hot water into a smooth paste. Add the vinegar, sugar, salt, soy sauce, and sesame oil. Mix thoroughly. Add the cabbage 1 cup at a time, mixing well after each addition. Sprinkle with cayenne to taste, and mix. Cover and refrigerate for at least 4 hours or up to 24 hours. Stir several times while chilling. Sprinkle with the crushed peanuts and chopped green onions just before serving.

The Hot Flash Cookbook

WAKAME AND BEAN SALAD

Makes 4 servings

This delicious deep-green seaweed salad combines white beans, crunchy radishes, and toasted hazelnuts in a mosaic of unusual tastes. An added plus: It is rich in iron and calcium.

4 ounces wakame (½ cup)

2 cups water

One 15-ounce can cannellini beans, rinsed and drained

1 cup thinly sliced radishes

3 tablespoons plain rice vinegar or white wine vinegar

1 tablespoon mirin (sweet sake) or dry sherry

1 tablespoon Dijon mustard

2 tablespoons Asian sesame oil

Freshly ground pepper to taste

¼ cup hazelnuts, toasted, peeled, and crushed (see page 52)

Soak the wakame in the water for about 15 minutes. Drain, remove and discard the tough ribs, and cut the tender parts into ½-inch squares. Combine with the beans and radishes in a large bowl and set aside.

In a small bowl, whisk together the vinegar, mirin or sherry, mustard, oil, and black pepper. Toss with the beans, radishes, and wakame. Sprinkle with the toasted hazelnuts.

VEGETARIAN

MAIN

DISHES

Yams and Cashew Curry

Makes 8 to 10 servings

The slightly nutty flavor of basmati rice is perfect with this hearty curry, which combines yams, red onions, potatoes, red peppers, and cashews, and is rich in mood-soothing potassium.

2 yams, peeled and cut into rounds,
  then into quarters

4 tablespoons olive oil

1 teaspoon minced fresh ginger

½ teaspoon yellow or brown mustard seed

3 to 4 garlic cloves, crushed

2 cups sliced red onions

1½ teaspoons salt

2 small potatoes, peeled and thinly sliced

½ teaspoon minced fennel frond

1 tablespoon ground cumin

1 teaspoon ground coriander

1 teaspoon dried dill weed

1 teaspoon ground turmeric

1½ cups orange juice

½ cup fresh lemon or lime juice

Cayenne pepper to taste

2 red bell peppers, seeded, deribbed,
   and thinly sliced

1½ cups (6 ounces) toasted cashew pieces

1 cup plain nonfat yogurt

Steamed basmati rice for serving

In a medium saucepan of boiling water, cook the yams until tender, about 4 minutes.

Heat the oil in a large skillet over medium heat. Add the ginger, mustard seeds, and garlic and sauté until the seeds split and pop, about 3 to 5 minutes.

Add the red onions, salt, potatoes, yams, minced fennel, herbs, and turmeric. Sauté for 5 to 7 minutes.

Add the orange juice and lemon or lime juice. Cover, reduce heat to medium low, and simmer until the potatoes are tender, about 10 to 15 minutes.

Add the cayenne and bell peppers, then the cashews. Cover and simmer briefly, about 1 minute. Remove from heat and stir in the yogurt. Serve with basmati rice.

Ruby Corn Pudding

Makes 6 servings

Serve this dish as a dramatically different main course or a brightly hued side dish. Ruby-red chard, full of vitamin A, melds creamily with red peppers to make a dish unique in both color and taste.

RUBY SAUCE	1 bunch beet greens with stems
	1 garlic clove, minced
	½ cup chopped green onion
	1 red jalapeño chile, diced
	1 cup nonfat chicken broth
	2 red bell peppers, roasted, peeled, seeded, and diced (see page 59)
	1 teaspoon minced canned chipotle chile en adobo
	Salt and freshly ground pepper to taste

CORN PUDDING	2 cups fresh creamed corn
	1 cup cornmeal
	¼ cup olive oil
	2 tablespoons butter, melted
	1 cup buttermilk

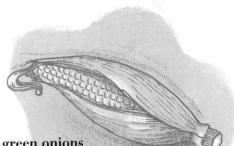

1 cup finely chopped green onions

½ cup fresh cilantro leaves, finely chopped

2 eggs, slightly beaten

½ cup (2 ounces) grated Parmesan cheese

3 Anaheim chiles, roasted, peeled,
  and diced (see page 59)

½ teaspoon baking soda

To prepare the ruby sauce: In a covered steamer or saucepan, steam the beet greens over boiling water for 7 minutes. Let cool and squeeze dry in a strainer. In a small saucepan, combine the garlic, green onions, jalapeño, and broth and bring to a boil. Reduce heat and simmer for 20 minutes. Transfer to a blender or food processor, add the beet greens, peppers, and chipotle, and puree until smooth. Add salt and pepper.

To prepare the corn pudding: Preheat the oven to 350°F. In a blender or food processor, puree the corn until creamy.

In a large bowl, combine the remaining ingredients. Stir in the corn puree until blended. Pour the batter into an oiled 8-cup casserole or baking dish. Bake for 1 hour, or until slightly browned and set. Cut into wedges and serve hot with the ruby sauce.

ROASTED FENNEL PARMESAN
ON SPINACH BED

Makes 6 servings

Roast, toast, and sweeten the fennel, then serve on a leafy spinach bed. Softly warmed spinach preserves its store of vitamin E, to improve circulation and protect the heart.

3 fennel bulbs, trimmed

3 tablespoons extra-virgin olive oil

2 tablespoons minced fresh marjoram and/or thyme

Salt and freshly ground pepper to taste

1 bunch fresh spinach, stemmed and shredded

¼ cup plain rice vinegar

3 tablespoons fresh lime juice

¼ cup grated Parmesan cheese

Halve the fennel bulbs from top to bottom, then cut each half into 3 or 4 wedges. In a baking dish large enough to hold the fennel, combine the oil, herbs, salt and pepper. Add the fennel and thoroughly coat with the oil mixture.

Toss the spinach with the vinegar and lime, then divide among 6 plates and set aside.

Preheat the oven to 400°F. Bake the fennel for about 40 minutes, or until tender. Sprinkle with the cheese and return to the oven until the cheese is melted and slightly brown. Top the spinach with the baked fennel and serve.

CITRUS-SPIKED CHARD

Serves 4

Chard is strong in flavor, rich in vitamin A and magnesium, and a tasty base for a sprinkling of sesame seeds.

> 1½ pounds Swiss chard, chopped
>
> Juice of 1 lemon
>
> Steamed rice or cooked pasta for serving
>
> ⅓ cup sesame seeds, toasted (see page 55)
>
> 1 teaspoon minced lemon pulp (see page 45)

In a covered steamer or saucepan, steam the greens over boiling water until just wilted, about 2 minutes. Immediately drizzle with the lemon juice so the leaves will retain their color. Serve over rice or pasta and garnish with sesame seeds and lemon pulp.

ASPARAGUS WITH
ROASTED RED PEPPER SAUCE

Makes 4 main-dish or 6 appetizer servings

Tender green asparagus blends perfectly with the smoky presence of roasted red pepper sauce.

1 garlic bulb

1 tablespoon olive oil

4 red bell peppers, seeded, deribbed, and chopped

½ teaspoon cayenne pepper

2 tablespoons soy sauce

2 tablespoons *each* lemon and orange juice

1 pound asparagus, trimmed

Preheat the oven to 350°F. Remove the papery outer husk of the garlic bulb. Place the garlic bulb in a small casserole. Drizzle with 2 tablespoons olive oil. Bake for about 45 minutes, or until very soft, turning the bulb once or twice during baking. Press the garlic out of the skins to make ½ cup roasted garlic. Puree the garlic in a blender or food processor and set aside.

Heat the oil in a large skillet over medium-high heat and sauté the peppers and cayenne for 2 minutes. Add the soy sauce and citrus juices and simmer for 2 more minutes, then transfer to blender or food processor and blend with the garlic puree.

In a covered steamer or saucepan, steam the asparagus over boiling water for 2 minutes, or until crisp-tender and bright green in color. Arrange the asparagus on a serving platter and drizzle with spirals of sauce.

BEANS AND BITTER GREENS

Makes 2 servings

This warm salad by Linda Hillel is rich in vitamin E, protein, and potassium. Try it for lunch on a cold day or as a light supper dish.

2 tablespoons extra-virgin olive oil

1 bunch dandelion, mustard, or turnip greens (10 to 12 ounces), stemmed and cut into ½-inch ribbons

4 garlic cloves, thinly sliced

2 tablespoons mirin (sweet sake) or dry sherry

2 tablespoons fresh lemon juice

1 tablespoon Dijon mustard

½ cup cooked garbanzo beans, drained and rinsed

¼ cup finely slivered red bell pepper or diced fresh tomato

Salt and freshly ground pepper to taste

In a large skillet or sauté pan, heat 1 tablespoon of the oil over medium-high heat. Add the greens and garlic and sauté for 1 minute. Lower heat, add the mirin or dry sherry, cover, and simmer for 10 minutes. Remove from heat.

In a small bowl, whisk together the lemon juice, mustard, and remaining 1 tablespoon oil. Add to the greens along with all the remaining ingredients. Toss thoroughly.

WHITE BEANS WITH CURRY SAUCE
AND GLAZED CARROTS

Makes 6 servings

Brimming with potassium, beans are a high-fiber, filling food that is digested slowly, thus calming and regulating the blood sugar level while adding a slight amount of vitamin E.

1 pound dried white beans

6 cups water

½ teaspoon cayenne pepper

1 garlic clove

1 teaspoon minced lemon pulp and membrane (see page 45)

1 bay leaf

2 teaspoons salt

GLAZED CARROTS

2 carrots, peeled

1 cup water

¼ cup sugar

CURRY SAUCE

2 tablespoons olive oil

1 large yellow onion, chopped

¼ cup minced celery leaves or fennel fronds

4 tablespoons curry powder

2 tablespoons flour

1 teaspoon minced fresh thyme, or ¼ teaspoon dried thyme

1 cup nonfat chicken broth

1 cup silken tofu

Juice of 1 lemon

Salt and freshly ground pepper to taste

2 teaspoons brandy

½ cup plain nonfat yogurt

Rinse and pick over the beans to remove any stones. Put the beans in a large bowl, cover with cold water, and let soak overnight. Drain and pour into a heavy 6-quart kettle. Add the water, cayenne, garlic, pulp and membrane, and bay leaf. Bring to a boil, reduce heat to a simmer, cover, and cook for 2 hours, or until tender. Add the salt the last 15 minutes of cooking and stir several times during cooking. Drain and set aside.

To make the glazed carrots: Using a very sharp vegetable peeler, cut long, ½-inch-wide paper-thin carrot slices.

Combine the water and sugar in a heavy saucepan. Bring to a boil, reduce heat to a simmer, and add the carrot strips. Cook until the carrots are tender and liquid has become a thick glaze, about 4 minutes. Let the carrots cool in the syrup.

To make the curry sauce: In a medium saucepan, heat the oil over medium heat. Add the onion and celery or fennel and cook for 5 minutes, or until the onion is translucent. Add the curry, flour, thyme, and broth. Lower heat and simmer for 5 minutes. Add the tofu, lemon juice, salt, pepper, and brandy. Strain through a fine-meshed sieve.

Add the yogurt and spoon over the beans. Garnish with the carrots and serve.

ORANGE-SCENTED CRANBERRY BEANS

Makes 4 servings

Fresh red-striped cream-colored cranberry shell beans are available in summer. Here they are flavored with orange zest, spices, and a puree of nuts and ginger.

10 whole cashew nuts

2 garlic cloves

One ½-inch piece fresh ginger, chopped

2 cups water

1 teaspoon olive oil

1 small jalapeño chile, seeded and minced

1 teaspoon ground coriander

½ teaspoon ground cumin

1¼ pounds fresh cranberry beans, shelled (2 cups)

1½ teaspoons grated orange zest

1 teaspoon salt, or to taste

¼ teaspoon minced orange membrane and pulp (see page 45)

Chopped fresh basil or cilantro for garnish

Combine the nuts, garlic, and ginger in a blender or food processor. Add ½ cup of the water and blend to a smooth puree.

Heat the oil in a large saucepan over medium heat. Add the jalapeño and cook, stirring, for 5 minutes. Add the coriander and cumin. Cook, stirring, for 1 minute. Add the beans and cook, stirring constantly, for 2 to 3 minutes.

Stir in the nut mixture and cook for 3 to 4 minutes. Add the orange zest, remaining 1½ cups water, and salt. Simmer, covered, until beans are tender, about 15 minutes.

Stir in the orange membrane and pulp just before serving. Transfer to a heated serving dish, garnish with the basil or cilantro, and serve.

APRICOT RISOTTO WITH HAZELNUTS

Makes 6 to 8 servings

The most important component of any risotto is Arborio rice, blended in this recipe with a generous helping of mellow apricots. Arborio rice has an extra-creamy texture due to its high starch content and is readily available in most stores.

3 cups nonfat chicken broth

½ cup hazelnuts, toasted and peeled (see page 52)

2 tablespoons pure olive oil

1 large onion, finely diced

1 cup Arborio rice

½ cup dry white wine

¼ cup freshly grated Parmesan cheese

2 tablespoons buttermilk

½ cup dried apricots, finely diced

½ teaspoon freshly grated nutmeg

In a medium saucepan, bring the chicken broth to a simmer. Set aside and keep warm. Grind the hazelnuts to a powder in a nut grinder, blender, or food processor and set aside.

Heat the olive oil over low heat in a large, heavy skillet. Add the onion, cover, and cook until translucent, about 2 minutes. Do not let it brown. Add the rice to the skillet, stirring to coat with the oil, and sauté with the onion for about 5 minutes, or until browned. Gradually add the wine, stirring with a wooden spoon.

When the wine has been completely absorbed, add the broth ½ cup at a time, stirring occasionally and cooking over very low heat until the broth has been completely absorbed and the grains are dense yet creamy, about 30 to 35 minutes. Add the Parmesan and buttermilk. Combine thoroughly. Add the ground hazelnuts, apricots, and nutmeg.

Vegetarian Main Dishes

Baked Pasta Squares
with Green Sauce

Makes 8 to 10 servings

The leafy greens of spinach, turnip, mustard, or beet are replete with vitamin E, as well as savory flavors. These baked pasta squares make delicious appetizers.

6 ounces bow tie pasta or egg noodles

GREEN
SAUCE

1 pound mustard greens

4 garlic cloves, minced

½ teaspoon salt

1 cup nonfat chicken broth

1 cup canned tomatoes

½ cup water

**½ cup grated Parmesan, crumbled goat
or farmer's cheese, or low-fat ricotta**

1 cup plus 1 teaspoon milk

3 tablespoons butter

½ cup all-purpose flour

½ teaspoon ground nutmeg

½ teaspoon salt

1 tablespoon olive oil

3 garlic cloves, minced

2 egg whites

2 eggs

¼ cup minced fresh parsley

1 cup pecans or walnuts, toasted and crushed (see pages 52–53)

Preheat oven to 350°F. In a large pot of salted boiling water, cook the pasta for about 3 minutes. Remove, rinse, and drain. Set aside.

To make the green sauce: In a covered steamer or saucepan, steam the greens over boiling water until tender, about 4 minutes. Transfer to a blender or food processor and puree with the remaining sauce ingredients until smooth. Set aside.

Heat the 1 cup milk in a small saucepan over low heat, letting it simmer until ready to use. In a large saucepan, melt the butter over a medium-low heat until bubbly, sprinkle with the flour, and cook for 3 minutes, stirring constantly; do not let it brown. Gradually whisk in the hot milk; cook and continue to stir until thickened. Carefully pour the pureed greens into the milk mixture, stirring until smooth. Let cool and add the nutmeg and salt.

Heat the oil in a saucepan and sauté the garlic until browned, about 2 minutes.

In a medium bowl, beat the egg whites until foamy. In a small bowl, beat the eggs with the 1 teaspoon milk. Blend in the whites, then fold into the cooled pasta mixture. Add the garlic. Oil the sides and bottom of a 9-inch square casserole dish. Place the mixture in the dish and bake for 30 minutes, or until done.

Let cool to room temperature. Sprinkle with parsley and nuts as garnish and cut into 8 to 10 squares.

Mirin and Kombu Bake

Makes 6 servings

This hearty stew by Linda Hillel combines tofu, mushrooms, and squash with kombu, a seaweed delicacy available in most Asian markets.

One 10-inch piece kombu

1½ cups water

3 tablespoons mirin (sweet sake) or dry sherry

3 tablespoons low-salt soy sauce

1 tablespoon slivered fresh ginger

2 onions, cut into thin wedges

1 pound shiitake mushrooms, stemmed and sliced ½ inch thick

1 unpeeled small kabocha squash (about 2 pounds), seeded and cut into 1-inch cubes

4 ounces firm tofu, rinsed, drained, and cut into 1-inch cubes

reheat the oven to 400°F. In a medium bowl, soak the kombu in the water for 15 minutes, or until softened. Remove from water, reserving the liquid, and cut into slivers.

Combine the kombu soaking water with the mirin or sherry, soy sauce, and ginger. Set aside.

Place all the remaining ingredients, including the kombu, in a large baking dish and gently toss to distribute evenly. Pour the soy sauce mixture evenly over the vegetables.

Cover and bake for about 30 minutes. Gently toss the vegetables in the liquid. Uncover and bake another 30 to 40 minutes, or until the squash is tender, stirring the vegetables every 10 minutes or so.

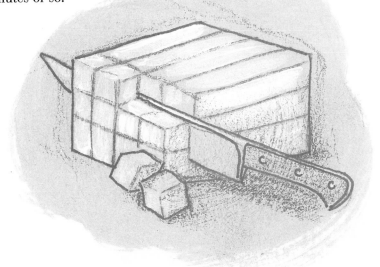

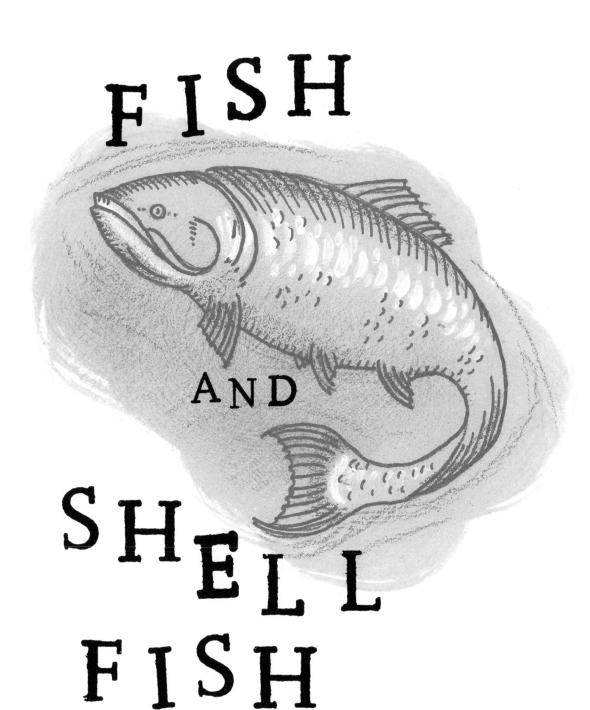

FISH

AND

SHELL
FISH

GRILLED SALMON
WITH TOMATILLO SAUCE

Makes 4 servings

The petite Mexican green tomato, or tomatillo, combines with the refreshing flavors of lemon and lime to make a tangy green sauce for grilled salmon fillets or steaks.

TOMATILLO
SAUCE

1¼ cups water

1 pound tomatillos, husked and quartered

1 tablespoon olive oil

1 corn tortilla

3 serrano chiles or 2 Anaheim chiles, stemmed and seeded

¼ cup chopped onion

¼ cup chopped fresh cilantro leaves

2 garlic cloves

1 teaspoon salt

1 teaspoon sugar

1 teaspoon cumin seeds, crushed

2 tablespoons fresh lime juice

4 salmon fillets or steaks, 6 to 8 ounces each

Salt and freshly ground pepper to taste

Juice of 1 lemon

¼ cup olive oil

1 tablespoon plain rice vinegar

To make the sauce: In a medium saucepan, bring 1 cup of the water to a boil. Add the tomatillos and cook for 6 minutes, or until tender. Remove from heat.

Heat the oil in a medium skillet over medium-high heat and fry the tortilla until crisp around the edges. Let cool slightly. Tear into pieces and put in a blender or food processor, along with the remaining ¼ cup water and all the remaining sauce ingredients. Puree to a smooth sauce.

Light a fire in a charcoal or gas grill. Remove the salmon from the refrigerator 30 minutes before serving. Season the salmon with salt and pepper. In a small bowl, mix the lemon, oil, and vinegar. Baste the salmon with the lemon mixture. Grill the salmon over medium-hot coals for 2 minutes on each side, or until almost opaque throughout; if cooking fillets, cook skin-side up, then turn. Serve with the tomatillo sauce.

King Mackerel Grill

Makes 4 servings

The firm, savory flesh of this fish is ideally suited for cubing and skewering. Often ignored because of a "high-fat" reputation, this fish has been reinstated as "king" due to its omega-3 oil content.

1 large mackerel, about 2 pounds

¼ cup olive oil

¼ cup fresh lemon juice

1 tablespoons anisette liqueur or Sambuca

1 garlic clove, crushed

Salt and freshly ground pepper to taste

5 to 7 bay leaves

1 fennel bulb with fronds

Steamed rice or couscous for serving

To prepare the fish: Cut the fish flesh away from the bone and cube it. Combine the oil, lemon juice, liqueur, garlic, salt, and pepper in a shallow nonaluminum container. Add the fish cubes and turn them to coat. Cover and refrigerate for at least 2 hours or overnight.

Light a fire in a charcoal or gas grill. Remove the fish from the refrigerator 30 minutes before cooking. Skewer the fish cubes with a bay leaf between each one.

Chop the fennel into sections, keeping the fronds intact. Soak the pieces in a bowl of water for 10 minutes.

When the coals are hot, drain the fennel and sprinkle it over the coals. Grill the fish for 3 minutes on each side. Serve immediately with rice or couscous.

POACHED MACKEREL
WITH SAFFRON-SPINACH SAUCE

Makes 4 servings

Behind its homespun demeanor, mackerel is one of the healthiest fin fish for midlife women, thanks to its heart-protecting omega-3 fatty acids. The following is an artful presentation of creamy white fish on a bed of deep green spinach.

2 tablespoons olive oil

1 tablespoon minced shallot

1 tablespoon flour

1¼ cups hot nonfat chicken broth

Pinch of saffron

½ bunch spinach (about 15 large leaves), stemmed and finely chopped

Sea salt and freshly ground pepper to taste

2 mackerel, salmon, or haddock fillets (about 1 pound)

2 tablespoons sour cream

Heat the olive oil in a large skillet or sauté pan over medium-low heat and cook the shallot for 3 minutes, or until translucent. Add the flour, stir until blended, and cook for 1 minute. Whisk in the broth, then stir in the saffron, spinach, salt, and pepper. Simmer, uncovered, for 3 to 4 minutes. Add the fish, cover, and cook gently just until fish flakes, 3 to 5 minutes. With a slotted metal spatula, transfer to a warm platter.

Stir the sour cream into the sauce until blended. Drizzle the sauce over or around fish.

Susan B. Trout with Sorrel Sauce

Makes 2 servings

The fresh appeal of trout is enhanced by a lemony bite of sorrel. Rainbow trout are high in linolenic acid, which helps the skin stay toned and supple.

2 rainbow trout fillets

2 tablespoons fresh lemon juice

3 tablespoons minced fennel fronds

SORREL SAUCE

2 sorrel leaves, stemmed

½ cup dry white wine

3 tablespoons fish stock or clam juice

1 cup pureed silken tofu

2 egg yolks

Salt, white pepper, and fresh lemon juice to taste

¼ teaspoon minced lemon pulp and membrane (see page 45)

reheat the broiler. Sprinkle each fillet with lemon juice and fennel. Broil for 2 to 3 minutes on each side, or until the fish begins to separate into flakes. Set aside and keep warm.

To make the sauce: Cut the sorrel leaves into thin strips and set aside. In a medium saucepan, combine the fish stock or clam juice and wine and bring to a boil. When just boiling, add half of the tofu and boil for 5 minutes. Set aside and keep warm.

Beat the egg yolks in a small bowl. Gradually whisk in $\frac{1}{2}$ cup of the hot liquid mixture. Add the egg yolk mixture to the remaining tofu and add to the mixture. Add the pulp and membrane.

Season with salt, pepper, and lemon juice. Add the sorrel leaves to the warm sauce and stir over medium heat for 1 minute. Pour over the trout and serve at once.

Fish and Vegetables in Parchment

Makes 4 servings

The mild, delicate flavor of sole is best preserved by steaming. Here, it is cooked in parchment with a variety of vitamin E-rich vegetables.

8 ounces spinach, stemmed and coarsely chopped

3 outer cabbage leaves

½ cup minced carrot leaves

½ cup snow peas

½ garlic clove

½ teaspoon minced fresh parsley

¼ teaspoon grated lemon zest

½ teaspoon minced lemon membrane and pulp (see page 45)

Olive oil for brushing

4 sole fillets

6 tablespoons dry white wine

Salt and freshly ground pepper to taste

Steamed rice for serving

Preheat the oven to 400°F. In a large bowl, combine the spinach, cabbage, carrot leaves, snow peas, garlic, parsley, and lemon zest, membrane, and pulp. Cut 4 pieces of baking parchment, aluminum foil, or waxed paper into rectangular shapes about twice the size of the fillets. Brush with oil. Place 1 fillet in the center of one half of each piece of parchment, foil, or paper along with one fourth of the vegetable mixture. Sprinkle with the white wine and salt and pepper. Fold the parchment, foil, or paper over the fish and seal each package by folding the edges down lunch-bag style. Place the packages on a baking sheet and bake for 8 to 10 minutes. Serve with steamed rice.

BLACKENED RED SNAPPER WITH MINT

Makes 6 servings

Bright cayenne pepper lends both spicy appeal and a healthy
dose of magnesium and bioflavonoids to this vibrant fish entree.
Peppermint leaves create an unusual flavor contrast and are rich
in vitamin E.

5 tablespoons canola oil

1 tablespoon sweet paprika

½ teaspoon onion powder

1 teaspoon cayenne pepper

½ teaspoon dried thyme

½ teaspoon dried oregano

½ teaspoon dried basil

¼ teaspoon ground cumin

½ teaspoon salt

¼ cup fresh mint leaves, minced

Six 5-ounce red snapper fillets,
    each about 1 inch thick

6 fresh lemon wedges

Fresh mint sprigs for garnish

Pour the oil into a shallow bowl. Combine the paprika, onion powder,
cayenne, thyme, oregano, basil, cumin, salt, and mint in another bowl, then
spread on a plate. Place a large cast-iron skillet over high heat until heated
throughout, about 2 minutes. Dip the fish in the oil, then coat both sides with
the spices and herbs. Cook the fish in batches if necessary, in the hot skillet on
one side for 1 minute, or until charred. Turn and blacken the other side. Garnish with lemon wedges and mint sprigs. Serve at once.

Spicy Pecan Halibut
with Asparagus

Makes 4 servings

A sprinkle of pecans crowns the king of the flatfishes in this savory dish. A glistening balsamic glaze adds full-bodied flavor.

SPICED
NUTS

1 tablespoon olive oil

½ cup pecan pieces, chopped

½ teaspoon cayenne pepper

½ teaspoon ground cumin

½ teaspoon salt

BALSAMIC
GLAZE

1 cup balsamic vinegar

2 tablespoons packed brown sugar

¼ teaspoon cayenne pepper

3 tablespoons pure olive oil

Four 8-ounce halibut steaks, each 1½ inches thick

Salt and freshly ground pepper to taste

2 teaspoons canola oil

1 pound baby asparagus spears, trimmed

To make the spiced nuts: In a small sauté pan or skillet, heat the oil over low heat. Add the pecans, cayenne, cumin, and salt and sauté until the nuts are lightly toasted. Set aside.

To make the glaze: Combine the vinegar, brown sugar, and cayenne in a small saucepan. Bring to a boil, reduce to a simmer, and cook to reduce to a thick glaze. Set aside.

Preheat the oven to 350°F. In a large skillet, heat the olive oil over high heat until almost smoking. Season the fish with salt and pepper and sear for 2 to 3 minutes on each side. Transfer the fish to a warm platter and set aside. In the same skillet, heat the canola oil over medium-high heat and sauté the asparagus, stirring constantly, for 3 to 4 minutes, or until crisp-tender.

To serve, drizzle the balsamic glaze over the fish, sprinkle with the spiced nuts, and garnish with a fan of asparagus.

Sea Bass Miso

Makes 4 servings

Miso is a delicious protein source that provides vitamin E as well. Here it combines with bass, daikon, ginger, and a sprinkle of soy to make a delightful Asian-flavored main course.

1 tablespoon sugar

1 tablespoon sake

½ cup white miso paste

2 pounds sea bass or salmon steaks

2 tablespoons low-salt soy sauce

Grated fresh ginger for garnish

Shaved daikon radish for garnish

In a small bowl, thoroughly combine the sugar, sake, and miso. Place the fish in a shallow nonaluminum container. Pour the miso mixture over the fish and turn to coat. Cover and refrigerate overnight.

Remove the fish from the refrigerator 30 minutes before cooking. Preheat the broiler. Drain the fish of excess marinade and broil for 5 to 8 minutes on each side. Transfer to a warm platter or plates. Sprinkle with soy sauce, fresh ginger, and shaved daikon. Serve at once.

Sweet and Sour Fish
with spicy blackberry sauce

Makes 4 servings

This variation on plum sauce uses blackberries to add spice as well as vitamin E to baked halibut.

SPICY
BLACKBERRY
SAUCE

1 teaspoon Asian sesame oil

1 onion, finely chopped

1¼ cups water

4 teaspoons low-salt soy sauce

1 tablespoon plain rice vinegar

2 cups fresh blackberries

1 teaspoon flour or cornstarch,
  dissolved in 2 teaspoons cold water (optional)

4 halibut steaks, about 8 ounces each

¼ teaspoon grated fresh ginger

½ teaspoon pepper

Preheat the oven to 350°F. **To make the sauce:** In a large skillet, heat the oil over medium-high heat and sauté the onion for 5 minutes. Add the water, soy sauce, rice vinegar, and blackberries. Bring to a boil and cook for 5 minutes, or until thickened. If still too thin, add the flour or cornstarch mixture, stir, and cook for 1 more minute, or until thickened.

Place the halibut in a baking pan. Cover with the blackberry sauce and bake for 25 minutes, or until flaky. Sprinkle with grated ginger and pepper.

Fish and Shellfish

SHRIMP AND CELERY SAUTÉ

Makes 2 servings

This sauté by Linda Hillel uses all parts of the celery, including the vitamin E-rich fronds of the outer leaf. Shrimp offer a delicious source of low-fat protein and "good" HDL cholesterol.

2 tablespoons olive oil

4 garlic cloves, minced

4 celery stalks, thinly sliced
   on diagonal (about 2½ cups)

½ cup chopped celery leaves

1 tablespoon celery seeds

8 ounces medium to large shrimp,
   peeled and deveined, tails left on

2 tablespoons mirin (sweet sake)
   or dry sherry

½ cup fresh or frozen peas

Salt and freshly ground pepper
   to taste

2 tablespoons fresh lemon juice

2 tablespoons minced fresh cilantro
   or parsley

2 tablespoons roasted peanuts,
   chopped (optional)

Heat the oil in a wok or a large skillet or sauté pan over medium heat. Add the garlic and celery stalks, leaves, and seeds. Sauté until just wilted, about 3 minutes. Add the shrimp and mirin or sherry. Cook for 1 minute, stirring constantly. Add the peas and cook another 1 to 2 minutes, or just until the shrimp turn pink and opaque. Add salt and pepper.

Place the shrimp mixture in a serving bowl or on a platter. Toss with the lemon juice and garnish with cilantro or parsley, and peanuts if desired.

Fettuccine with Oysters and Arugula

Makes 2 servings

Vitamin E-rich oysters make a luscious topping for fresh fettuccine
in this unusual dish by Linda Hillel. The rich undertone of
sesame oil flavors the sliced celery, capers, tomato, and oysters.

1 tablespoon vegetable oil

2 shallots, minced, or 1 small
  onion, finely chopped

3 garlic cloves, minced

2 celery stalks with leaves,
  thinly sliced on the diagonal

¼ cup dry white wine

One 10-ounce jar oysters,
  drained and juice reserved

1 small tomato, diced

1½ tablespoons capers, drained

¼ cup heavy cream or
  2 egg whites and 2 tablespoons
  milk, beaten separately, then
  milk added

Salt and freshly ground pepper
  to taste

1 bunch arugula,
  stemmed and coarsely chopped

12 ounces fresh fettuccine

¼ cup fresh minced parsley

Freshly grated Parmesan cheese
  for serving

In a large skillet, heat the oil over medium heat and sauté the shallots or onion
and garlic for 1 minute. Add the celery and sauté another 2 or 3 minutes. Add the
wine and reserved oyster juice, bring to a boil, then lower heat to a simmer. Add
the oysters, tomato, capers, cream or egg white mixture, salt, and pepper. Simmer
until all the ingredients are heated through. Stir in the arugula until wilted.

Cook the pasta in a large pot of salted boiling water until al dente, about 2
to 3 minutes; drain. Transfer to a warm serving bowl and toss with the sauce
and parsley. Serve with Parmesan cheese.

Fish and Shellfish

GRILLED SHRIMP
WITH MUSTARD GREEN SALSA

Makes 2 main-dish or 4 to 6 appetizer servings

Spicy mustard greens and tangy lemon dress up grilled shrimp for an appetizer or main course. Enjoy the savory, unusual tang of mustard greens as well as their vivid color.

1 pound large shrimp, peeled and deveined, tails left on

4 tablespoons extra-virgin olive oil

Freshly ground pepper to taste

1 tablespoon mustard seeds

1 pound mustard greens, stemmed and coarsely chopped

4 garlic cloves, chopped

½ cup fresh lemon juice

1 tablespoon grated lemon zest

2 tablespoons Dijon mustard

¼ cup low-fat mayonnaise

Salt to taste

Lemon zest curls for garnish

ight a fire in a gas or charcoal grill. In a medium bowl, toss the shrimp with 1 tablespoon of the oil and the pepper. Set aside.

In a sauté pan, sauté the mustard seeds over medium-high heat until fragrant, stirring constantly. Transfer to a bowl and set aside. Add 1 tablespoon of the oil to the pan and sauté the mustard greens over medium heat until wilted, about 5 minutes. Add the garlic and cook 1 more minute.

Transfer the greens to a blender or food processor. Add the lemon juice and zest, mustard, mayonnaise, salt, and pepper to taste. Blend until smooth.

Place the shrimp in a small bowl, add the remaining 2 tablespoons oil, and toss until lightly coated. Skewer the shrimp and grill over white-hot coals until pink and opaque, 1 to 2 minutes per side.

Spoon the salsa in the center of each serving plate and surround with shrimp. Top each shrimp with a lemon zest curl.

POULTRY AND MEATS

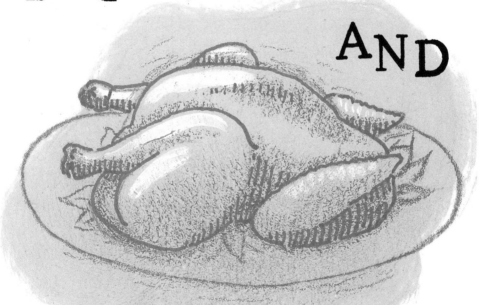

GRILLED LEMON-GARLIC CHICKEN

Makes 4 servings

Linda Hillel's recipe for a well-dressed chicken melds lemon, mustard, garlic, and black pepper into a simple yet savory dish. Tangy lemon is rich in flavonoids, while garlic boosts the good (HDL) cholesterol.

1 teaspoon grated lemon zest

⅓ cup freshly squeezed lemon juice

¼ cup extra-virgin olive oil

2 tablespoons Dijon mustard

Freshly ground pepper to taste

2 garlic cloves, pressed

4 skinless, boneless chicken breast halves

10 to 12 ounces spinach, stemmed and coarsely chopped

Nasturtium blossoms and/or slivered yellow bell peppers for garnish n a small bowl, whisk together the lemon zest, juice, oil, mustard, and pepper. Pour about two thirds of the mixture into a bowl large enough to hold the chicken. Reserve the remaining dressing.

Add the garlic to the bowl, then add the chicken and toss to coat. Cover and marinate for 1 hour at room temperature, or refrigerate for 2 to 24 hours.

Light a fire in a charcoal or gas grill. If the chicken has been refrigerated, remove it from the refrigerator 30 minutes before cooking. Cook the chicken over a medium-hot fire for 3 to 4 minutes per side, or until opaque throughout.

Meanwhile, in a covered steamer or saucepan, steam the spinach over boiling water just until wilted, about 1 minute. Toss with the reserved dressing.

Divide the spinach among 4 dinner plates and top with a chicken breast half. Garnish with nasturtiums and/or yellow bell pepper slivers.

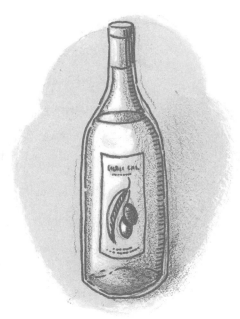

Poultry and Meats

Calico Chicken with Ginger

Makes 6 servings

Succulent vegetables in colorful medley are coated with a rich,
spicy nectar of ginger, garlic, soy, and sesame oil, which contains
essential fats and heart-protecting vitamin E.

CHICKEN

3 tablespoons olive oil

6 chicken thighs, skinned

2 garlic cloves, minced

6 tablespoons low-salt soy sauce

¼ cup dry red wine

3 tablespoons packed brown sugar

DRESSING

2 tablespoons grated fresh ginger

¼ cup low-salt soy sauce

2 tablespoons mirin or dry sherry (optional)

1 teaspoon minced garlic

1 teaspoon Asian sesame oil

1 teaspoon chili oil, or ½ teaspoon red pepper flakes

2 whole scallions, minced

2 tablespoons fresh lemon juice

¼ cup orange juice

3 teaspoons minced orange pulp and membrane
(see page 45)

The Hot Flash Cookbook

VEGETABLES 1 carrot, peeled and cut into ¼-inch rounds

1 zucchini, cut into ¼-inch rounds

1 fennel bulb, trimmed and cut into ¼-inch-thick lengthwise slices

8 ounces snow peas

4 ounces asparagus, cut into ¼-inch pieces

2 tablespoons olive oil

1 *each* large red and yellow bell pepper, seeded, deribbed, and cut into julienne

4 sorrel leaves, cut into shreds

Grated zest of 1 lemon

Salt and freshly ground pepper to taste

Steamed brown rice for serving

To prepare the chicken: In a large sauté pan or skillet, heat the oil over medium-high heat. Add the chicken thighs. Cook for 5 minutes, then turn. Cover the pan and cook for 10 minutes. Add garlic and sauté for 1 minute. Add the soy sauce, wine, and sugar and cook, uncovered, until the liquid has thickened. Turn the thighs, cover, and cook 5 minutes. Remove from heat, keeping the skillet covered.

To make the dressing: Combine all the ingredients in a saucepan and bring to a boil. Reduce heat and simmer for 5 minutes. Remove from heat and set aside.

To prepare the vegetables: In a large pot of boiling water, blanch the carrot for 2 minutes. Add the zucchini and cook for 1 minute. Add the fennel, snow peas, and asparagus. Cook for 1 minute. Drain the vegetables and rinse briefly under cold water.

In a large skillet, heat the oil over medium-high heat and sauté the pepper strips for 3 minutes. Add the blanched vegetables, sorrel, and zest. Add salt and pepper.

Arrange the chicken on a bed of brown rice, drizzle with the ginger dressing, and fan the vegetables alongside.

Note: Because the pulp and membrane are slightly bitter, the dressing must be used within several hours.

BLACKBERRY CHICKEN

Makes 4 servings

Rich, dark berries make a dramatic, savory sauce for sautéed chicken in this summery entree.

2 boneless, skinless whole chicken breasts

2 tablespoons olive oil

2 tablespoons minced shallots

¼ cup blackberry vinegar or white wine vinegar

¼ cup nonfat chicken broth

1 tablespoon blackberry brandy

1 cup fresh blackberries

2 tablespoons plain nonfat yogurt

2 tablespoons pureed soft tofu

Fresh chervil leaves for garnish

Rinse the chicken and pat dry with paper towels. Flatten each breast with the flat end of a meat pounder until about ½ inch thick, then cut into ½-inch-wide strips. In a large sauté pan or skillet, heat the oil over medium heat. Add the chicken and cook until lightly colored, about 3 to 6 minutes. Using tongs, remove from the skillet and set aside.

Add the shallots to the skillet and cook over low heat until translucent, 4 to 6 minutes. Add the vinegar, raise the heat to medium, and cook, stirring occasionally, until reduced to a thick syrup. Whisk in the broth and brandy. Simmer for 1 minute.

Return the chicken strips to the skillet and simmer gently in the sauce for about 5 minutes. Arrange the strips on a heated serving platter.

Simmer the sauce gently until it has further reduced and thickened slightly, about 3 minutes. Add the blackberries and cook for 1 minute. Remove from heat and gently stir in the yogurt and tofu. Pour the sauce over the chicken strips, garnish with chervil leaves, and serve at once.

GAME HENS WITH WILD RICE
AND ORANGE-GINGER GLAZE

Makes 4 servings

Plump hens gleam with orange sauce in this ginger-rich recipe by Linda Hillel.

ORANGE-
GINGER GLAZE

2 tablespoons unsalted butter

2 garlic cloves, pressed

2 tablespoons packed brown sugar

4 teaspoons ground ginger

½ cup fresh orange juice

3 tablespoons low-salt soy sauce

2 tablespoons mirin (sweet sake) or dry sherry

4 game hens

1 cup wild rice

1 onion, chopped

¼ cup chopped fennel fronds

½ fennel bulb, finely chopped

5 ounces chopped fresh mushrooms (any variety)

Grated zest of 1 orange

The Hot Flash Cookbook

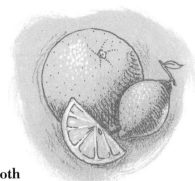

4 cups nonfat chicken broth

Salt and freshly ground pepper to taste

Orange zest curls for garnish

To make the glaze: Melt the butter in a small saucepan over low heat. Add the remaining glaze ingredients. Cook, stirring constantly, for 3 minutes. Do not boil. Let cool for 5 minutes.

Wash the hens, pat dry, and place in a bowl. Pour the warm glaze over the hens to coat. Set aside.

Rinse the wild rice and put it in a heavy, medium saucepan with all the remaining ingredients except the zest curls. Bring to a boil, cover, reduce heat to low, and cook until the rice is tender and the liquid is absorbed, about 40 minutes.

Preheat the oven to 450°F. Stuff each hen with about ¾ cup rice. Place the hens on a rack in a roasting pan and bake for about 40 minutes, or until the juices run clear. Baste with the glaze several times during baking. Remove, let cool slightly, and serve garnished with orange curls. Reheat and serve the remaining wild rice on the side.

GRILLED LAMB TENDERLOIN
WITH FENNEL GREMOLATA

Makes 4 to 6 servings

Tender lamb is even more delectable with the intense mint and fennel zing of this gremolata. Lamb is also rich in vitamin E.

MARINADE
½ cup olive oil

¼ cup dry white wine

¼ cup orange juice

1 teaspoon grated orange zest

1 tablespoon pepper

One 3-pound lamb tenderloin

GREMOLATA
½ fennel bulb, stemmed and cut into crosswise slices (fronds reserved)

1 cup minced fresh mint leaves

1 cup minced fresh parsley

1 garlic clove, minced

2 tablespoons grated lemon zest

2 tablespoons fresh lemon juice

6 tablespoons mint jelly

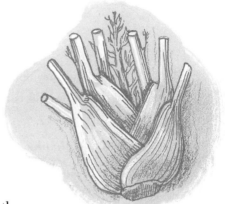

To make the marinade: Combine all the ingredients in a large nonaluminum baking pan. Add the lamb, cover, and refrigerate overnight or up to 2 days, turning occasionally.

To make the gremolata: In a small saucepan of boiling water, blanch the fennel pieces for 1 minute; drain. Combine the fennel and all the remaining ingredients in a medium bowl and let sit for at least 30 minutes. To store, cover and refrigerate for up to 1 week.

Remove the lamb from the refrigerator 30 minutes before cooking. Light a fire in a charcoal grill. Grill over a hot fire, basting frequently with the marinade, for 2 minutes on each side for medium rare.

Serve the lamb topped with the gremolata. Garnish with sprays of reserved fennel fronds.

Braised Lamb Shanks
WITH PARSLEY-PERSIMMON SAUCE

Makes 6 servings

Orange, nutmeg, and bay lend a hearty harvest touch to this succulent lamb dish, which is rich in vitamins A and E.

6 lamb shanks (about 1 pound each)

3 tablespoons olive oil

4 onions, halved lengthwise and cut crosswise into ¼-inch-thick slices

4 large garlic cloves, minced

4 cups water

1 bay leaf

2 cinnamon sticks

⅛ teaspoon ground cardamom

⅛ teaspoon ground nutmeg

½ teaspoon grated orange zest

Salt and freshly ground black pepper to taste

PARSLEY-PERSIMMON SAUCE

1 tablespoon olive oil

1 garlic clove, crushed

½ teaspoon sugar

¼ cup water

2 tablespoons flour

1 cup blood orange juice

½ ripe Fuyu persimmon, seeded and mashed

½ cup coarsely chopped fresh Italian parsley

½ teaspoon fennel seeds

¼ teaspoon salt

¼ teaspoon pepper

Preheat the oven to 350°F. Pat the lamb shanks dry. In a large cast-iron skillet, heat 2 tablespoons of the oil over medium-high heat and brown the lamb shanks on all sides. Transfer the lamb to a Dutch oven. Pour off the fat from the skillet.

Heat the remaining 1 tablespoon oil in the same skillet over medium heat. Add the onions and garlic to the skillet and sauté until golden. Add to the lamb, then add all the remaining ingredients. Bring the liquid to a boil. Cover and braise in the oven until just tender, about 1¾ hours.

To make the sauce: In a medium saucepan, heat the oil over medium-high heat. Add the garlic and cook for 30 seconds. Reduce heat to medium low, add the sugar, water, and flour, and mix until thickened. Gradually add the orange juice, stirring constantly. Add the persimmon, parsley, fennel seeds, salt, and pepper. Set aside and keep warm. Serve on the side with the lamb shanks.

Lamb and Sweet Potato Curry

Makes 4 servings

This tasty curry of cumin-spiced vegetables and lamb has the added richness of yogurt. Enjoy sweet potatoes, rich in vitamin A and potassium.

> 2 teaspoons olive oil
>
> 12 ounces boneless lamb sirloin, trimmed and cut into ½-inch-thick pieces
>
> 1 cup chopped onion
>
> 2 garlic cloves, chopped
>
> One 16-ounce can whole tomatoes
>
> 1 pound red-skinned sweet potatoes (yams), peeled and cubed
>
> 8 ounces green beans, cut into 1-inch lengths
>
> 1½ teaspoons ground cumin
>
> Salt and freshly ground pepper to taste
>
> 1 cup plain nonfat yogurt
>
> Chopped fresh cilantro for garnish

In a large skillet, heat the oil over high heat and sauté the lamb for 2 minutes. Reduce heat to medium and add the onion, garlic, tomatoes, potatoes, beans, and cumin. Simmer until tender, about 15 minutes. Add salt and pepper. Serve topped with yogurt and cilantro.

LAMB ON A BED OF LEEKS

Makes 4 to 6 servings

Vitamin E-bearing lamb and leeks are served with a tart juniper berry and orange sauce.

1 teaspoon unsalted butter

1 garlic clove, crushed

½ cup coarsely chopped
   fresh parsley

½ teaspoon fennel seeds

½ teaspoon sugar

¼ teaspoon pepper

¼ cup fresh blood orange juice

3 juniper berries, crushed

2 leeks, including ½ inch of the
   green, washed and cut into fine
   julienne strips

1 tablespoon olive oil

1 pound cooked lamb shoulder, leg,
   or loin, cut into small strips

1 large outer leaf Napa or
   red cabbage, shredded

2 blood oranges, sliced

In a medium sauté pan or skillet, melt the butter over medium-high heat and sauté the garlic and parsley for 1 to 2 minutes. Add the seeds, sugar, pepper, and orange juice. Cook for 2 minutes, or until slightly thickened. Add the juniper berries and leeks. Stir, cover, and cook for 3 minutes, or until crisp-tender. Using a slotted spoon, transfer the leeks to a bowl and keep warm.

Add the oil to the same pan. Over high heat, bring the liquid in the pan to a boil. Add the lamb, turning to coat completely. Reduce heat to medium and cook until the liquid is almost evaporated.

Make a bed of leeks on each serving plate. Sprinkle the cabbage over the leeks. Fan the orange slices around the leeks. Top with the lamb and serve.

Beef Fajitas with Balsamic Glaze

Makes 2 servings

A tasty touch of the Southwest, these jalapeño-spiced beef strips are given an added flavor boost with a sweet-spicy glaze.

12 ounces ½-inch-thick boneless sirloin steak

1 teaspoon sesame seeds

½ teaspoon whole cumin seeds, crushed

2 teaspoons olive oil

3 garlic cloves, minced

½ jalapeño chile, minced

3 tablespoons mirin (sweet sake) or dry sherry

1 tablespoon low-salt soy sauce

3 teaspoons balsamic vinegar

1 teaspoon packed brown sugar

⅛ teaspoon cayenne pepper

Warm flour tortillas

lice the steak into thin strips. Sprinkle with sesame and cumin seeds. In a large, heavy skillet, heat the oil over medium-high heat until almost smoking. Add the meat strips and sauté for 3 minutes for medium-rare fajitas. Transfer to a small platter and keep warm.

Pour off any fat from the skillet. Add the garlic and jalapeño, and sauté for 10 seconds. Add the mirin or sherry and cook until almost all the liquid is evaporated. Remove from heat and add the soy sauce, vinegar, brown sugar, and cayenne. Return to low heat and simmer, stirring constantly, for 5 minutes until mixed. Add the meat strips and toss to coat. Divide among the tortillas and serve at once.

SIDE

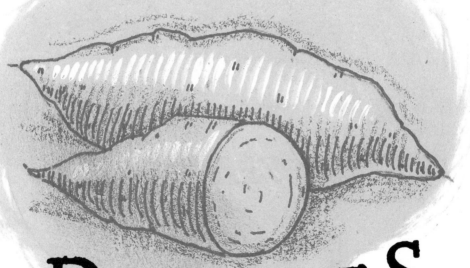

DISHES

Asparagus with Asafetida

Makes 4 servings

North Indian roasting spices include asafetida, the powdered dried sap of the giant fennel plant, which simmers into a mellow, garlicky flavor that complements fresh asparagus.

> **1 bunch asparagus (about 1 pound), trimmed**
>
> **2 tablespoons Asian sesame oil or wheat germ oil**
>
> **1½ teaspoons ground cumin**
>
> **½ teaspoon asafetida powder
> (available in Indian markets)**
>
> **½ teaspoon salt**
>
> **1 teaspoon honey**
>
> **1 teaspoon mango powder *(amchoor)*,
> available in Indian markets**
>
> **3 tablespoons fresh lime juice**

In a covered steamer or saucepan, steam the asparagus over boiling water until crisp-tender, about 2 minutes. Plunge it into cold water to stop the cooking; drain and set aside.

In a large skillet or sauté pan over medium-high heat, heat the oil. Add the cumin, asafetida, salt, honey, and mango powder and cook for several seconds. Add the asparagus and stir-fry until each stalk is completely coated. Drizzle with lime juice and serve immediately.

Marinated Carrots with Garlic

Makes 6 servings

Flavorful garlic lends an Algerian touch to this nutritious dish by Lalia Mohamed. Serve as a picnic dish, snack, or salad.

6 to 8 garlic cloves, crushed

1 teaspoon ground cumin

1 teaspoon paprika

1 teaspoon salt

2 tablespoons plus ⅓ cup water

2 tablespoons olive oil

6 carrots, peeled and cut into
    ¼-inch-thick slices (3½ cups)

⅓ cup minced fresh cilantro

Combine the garlic, spices, and salt in a small bowl. Add the 2 tablespoons water and mix thoroughly.

In a heavy, medium saucepan over medium-high heat, heat the olive oil. Add the garlic mixture and sauté about 30 seconds. Stir in the carrots and cilantro. Pour the ⅓ cup water over the carrots. Cover and cook over low heat for 15 to 20 minutes, or until crisp-tender. Uncover the pan and cook over high heat until all the juices evaporate. Transfer to a bowl and let cool to room temperature before serving.

Fennel in Cream Sauce

Makes 4 servings

A savory use of the entire fennel plant—seeds, stalk, and fronds—
in this creamy baked side dish. A perfect companion to steamed
fish.

CREAM
SAUCE

2 cups diced yellow onions

3 garlic cloves

½ cup silken tofu

¾ cup water

¼ teaspoon salt

¼ teaspoon white pepper

½ teaspoon prepared horseradish

½ teaspoon flour

2 fennel bulbs (1 pound)

2 tablespoons flour

1 tablespoon fennel seeds

¼ cup dried bread crumbs

To make the cream sauce: In a covered steamer or saucepan, steam the onions and garlic over boiling water until tender, about 2 minutes. Transfer to a blender or food processor and puree until smooth. Return the puree to the pan and add the tofu, ½ cup of the water, the salt, pepper, and horseradish. Simmer over low heat for 10 minutes.

In a medium bowl, dissolve the flour in the remaining ¼ cup water. Whisk half the simmering onion puree into the flour mixture and stir until smooth. Gradually whisk the liquid into the onion puree. Simmer for 15 minutes.

Cut the fennel bulbs and stems into ¼-inch-thick pieces and toss with the flour in a large bowl. Reserve the fennel fronds for garnish.

Heat a dry skillet over medium-high heat. Add the fennel seeds, toast for 30 seconds, and sprinkle them over the fennel. Put the floured fennel in a lightly oiled casserole dish. Pour the sauce over until it covers the fennel. Top with the bread crumbs and bake for 30 minutes.

Chop the fennel fronds and sprinkle them over the dish. Serve hot.

Fennel with Roasted Red Peppers

A visual and culinary treat, cool green fennel contrasts with sweet red peppers and vivid cayenne in this dish. Serve with steamed rice or pasta. To increase vigor, counteract fatigue.

3 fennel bulbs, trimmed and thinly sliced, fronds reserved

2 tablespoons fennel seed, crushed

¾ teaspoon cumin seed, crushed

Cayenne pepper or red pepper flakes to taste

1 teaspoon fresh lemon juice

1 tablespoon grated orange zest

3 tablespoons orange juice

1 small garlic clove, minced

3 tablespoons extra-virgin olive oil

2 teaspoons salt

Freshly ground pepper to taste

2 red bell peppers, roasted, peeled, and cut into thin slices (see page 59)

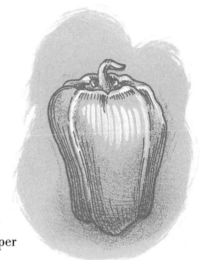

In a medium bowl, toss the fennel with the fennel seed, cumin seed, and cayenne or pepper flakes.

In a small bowl, stir the lemon juice, orange zest and juice, garlic, oil, salt, and pepper together. Pour over the fennel and let sit for 1 hour at room temperature.

Just before serving, add the red peppers. Mince the reserved fennel fronds and sprinkle over the vegetables.

Braised Fennel
WITH TOMATOES AND CAPERS

Makes 6 servings

A hearty, satisfying dish by Linda Hillel, featuring garlic-laced fennel bulbs simmered with tomatoes and thyme. Phytoestrogens in fennel mimic estrogen, and stimulate the cells.

3 fennel bulbs

¼ cup olive oil

3 garlic cloves, sliced

2 tomatoes, diced

¼ teaspoon dried thyme

2 tablespoons capers, drained

Salt and freshly ground black pepper to taste

Trim the fennel, reserving the fronds. Halve the fennel bulbs from top to bottom, then cut each half into thin wedges. In a large skillet or sauté pan over medium-high heat, heat the oil and sauté the fennel and garlic for 3 minutes. Add the tomatoes and thyme. Cover, lower heat, and simmer until the fennel is tender, about 15 minutes. Mince 2 tablespoons fennel fronds. Stir the capers and fennel fronds into the fennel. Cook, uncovered, for 2 minutes. Add the salt and pepper.

Mrs. Kale Gets Steamed

Makes 2 servings

Linda Hillel devised this tasty iron-rich dish of braised kale,
served on a bed of soba noodles and topped with toasted almonds.

1 bunch green or red kale, stemmed (reserve stems)

2 tablespoons canola oil

3 garlic cloves, chopped

⅓ cup low-salt vegetable broth or nonfat chicken broth

2 tablespoons low-fat soy sauce

2 tablespoons plain rice vinegar

1 tablespoon grated lemon zest

1 tablespoon fresh lemon juice

Freshly ground pepper to taste

10 ounces soba noodles

¼ cup slivered almonds, toasted (see pages 52–53)

2 tablespoons crumbled nori (optional)

Slice the kale stems thinly and chop the leaves coarsely. Heat the oil in a
large sauté pan or skillet over medium heat. Sauté the garlic and kale stems for
3 minutes. Add the kale leaves, broth, and soy sauce. Cover and cook until the
kale is tender, about 8 minutes. Remove from heat. Add the vinegar, lemon zest
and juice, and pepper and toss. Set aside and keep warm.

In a large pot of boiling water, cook the noodles until tender, about 2 minutes; drain. Serve the kale on a bed of noodles and top with the almonds and
nori, if desired.

Side Dishes

BROCCOLI BOUQUET

A festoon of green broccoli florets with leaves is dressed with mustard and tarragon. Broccoli's outer leaf is the most vitamin-rich part of the plant.

Florets from 2 bunches fresh broccoli with leaves

3 red bell peppers, seeded, deveined, and sliced into slivers

1 small bunch basil or fresh tarragon, stemmed and minced

1 cup plain nonfat yogurt

2 tablespoons Dijon mustard

¼ cup tarragon vinegar

⅔ cup olive oil

Salt and freshly ground pepper to taste

Place the florets in a covered steamer or saucepan and steam over boiling water until crisp-tender, about 2 minutes. Plunge them into ice water to cool, then drain. Combine with the red pepper.

Mince the broccoli leaves. Combine the minced leaves and basil or tarragon in a bowl and set aside.

Combine the yogurt, mustard, vinegar, oil, basil or tarragon mixture, salt, and pepper. Pour over the broccoli florets and red pepper slivers and toss.

Tamarind Mashed Yams

Makes 4 servings

Tasty, exotic, yet deeply satisfying in the homespun style of mashed potatoes, the yams are spiked with lemon, cumin, and tamarind. Adds magnesium for bone health, as well as vitamin E.

2 large yams (about 1½ pounds)

1 tablespoon olive oil

2 garlic cloves, minced

½ teaspoon cumin seeds, crushed

½ cup milk or buttermilk

1 teaspoon tamarind paste,
    dissolved in 1 teaspoon water

¼ teaspoon grated lemon zest

Minced fresh parsley for garnish

Scrub and pierce the yams with a fork. In a covered steamer or stockpot, steam the yams over boiling water until soft, about 20 minutes. Let cool to the touch.

In a small skillet over medium-high heat, heat the oil and sauté the garlic until it just begins to crisp, about 3 minutes. Remove from heat and set aside.

Scoop the flesh of the yams into a large bowl. Add the garlic, cumin seeds, milk or buttermilk, tamarind mixture, and lemon zest. With a large, heavy whisk, beat until mixture is creamy and soft. Serve garnished with parsley.

Balsamic-Glazed Yams

Makes 2 servings

Glazed yams elicit a double "yum," thanks to a rich glaze of sherry, soy sauce, balsamic vinegar, and spices.

> **2 yams, peeled and cut in half**
>
> **½ cup water**
>
> **6 tablespoons dry sherry**
>
> **2 tablespoons low-salt soy sauce**
>
> **4 tablespoons balsamic vinegar**
>
> **2 teaspoons honey**
>
> **Dash of ground cardamom**
>
> **Dash of ground cloves**
>
> **Dash of pepper**

Preheat the oven to 350°F. Combine the yams and water in a casserole. Cover and bake for 20 minutes. Remove the yams from the oven; drain, reserving the liquid.

In a large skillet, combine the yam liquid and sherry and bring to a boil. Cook until the liquid is almost evaporated. Add the soy sauce, vinegar, and honey. Lower heat to a simmer. Cook, stirring constantly, until thickened.

Finally, add the spices and yams. Spoon the glaze over the yams and cook for about 10 minutes, or until fork-tender.

Pumpkin Home Fries

Makes 6 servings

The earthy taste of toasted coriander seeds beautifully complements the smooth mellowness of pumpkin. Pumpkin, sesame seeds, and olive oil are all rich in vitamin E. Serve with baked fish or a vegetable casserole.

One ½ pound pumpkin, halved, seeded, peeled, and cut into ¼ -inch-thick slices

2 tablespoons olive oil

½ teaspoon salt

¼ teaspoon pepper

1 tablespoon sesame seeds, toasted (see page 55)

¾ teaspoon coriander seeds, toasted and crushed (see page 55)

Preheat the oven to 450°F. In a medium bowl, toss the pumpkin slices with the oil, salt, and pepper to coat evenly. Spread the pumpkin slices out in one layer on a baking sheet. Bake, turning occasionally, until the fries are browned and crisp outside and tender inside, about 20 minutes. Sprinkle with the sesame and coriander seeds before serving.

ROASTED BUTTERNUT SQUASH
WITH HAZELNUTS

Makes 4 servings

Squash and nuts, rich in vitamin E, make this delectable side dish
by Linda Hillel ideal for turkey or roast chicken.

1 butternut squash (1 to 1½ pounds)

Olive oil for brushing

Dash of freshly grated nutmeg

½ cup hazelnuts

Preheat the oven to 400°F. Cut the squash into quarters and remove the
seeds. Put the pieces in a baking dish, skin-side down. Brush the squash with
oil, sprinkle with nutmeg, and bake for about 1 hour, or until tender when
pierced with a fork.

While the squash is baking, toast the hazelnuts in a pie pan in the oven until
lightly browned, about 5 minutes. When the squash is done, rub the hazelnuts
briskly in a linen dish towel to remove the skins. Chop the nuts coarsely. Sprinkle the squash with the hazelnuts and serve hot.

SAUCES, SALSAS, AND CONDIMENTS

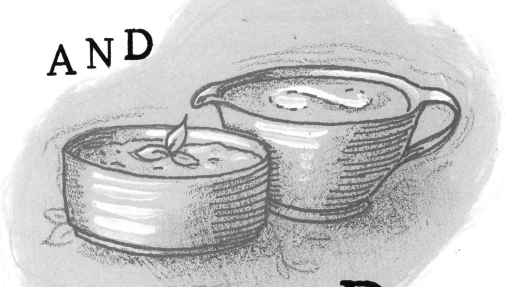

Mango Tango

Makes ¾ cup

This salsa is delicious drizzled over smoked chicken salad or on flavorful greens, like arugula.

1 ripe mango, peeled, pitted, and cut into cubes

2 tablespoons Asian sesame oil

2 tablespoons plain rice vinegar

½ teaspoon curry powder

⅛ teaspoon cumin seeds, crushed

Place all the ingredients in a blender or food processor and puree until smooth. Let sit for 30 minutes before using. Store in an airtight container in the refrigerator.

Blood Orange Vinaigrette

Makes about ⅞ cup

Tart blood oranges make a particularly delicious dressing for bean sprouts and mixed baby greens.

> ½ cup extra-virgin olive oil
>
> ¼ cup champagne vinegar
>
> 2 teaspoons grated blood orange zest
>
> 3 tablespoons blood orange juice
>
> 1 teaspoon minced blood orange membrane
>   and pulp (see page 45)
>
> Dash of white pepper

In a small bowl, whisk together all the ingredients. Pour into an airtight container, cover, and refrigerate until ready to serve.

YAM VINAIGRETTE

Makes about 1 cup

For decorative appeal, swirl this bright yellow puree on a plate, then half-cover with hot filled pasta and steamed vegetables.

> 1 small yam, peeled and cut into ½-inch chunks
>
> ½ cup orange juice
>
> ½ cup wheat germ oil or extra-virgin olive oil
>
> ¼ cup champagne vinegar
>
> 2 tablespoons seasoned rice vinegar
>
> 2 tablespoons Dijon mustard
>
> Salt and freshly ground pepper to taste

In a small saucepan of salted boiling water, cook the yam chunks until very tender, about 15 minutes; strain. Puree the yam and orange juice in a blender or food processor. With the machine running, gradually add the oil, vinegars, and mustard. Season with salt and pepper. Store in an airtight container in the refrigerator.

Anchovy-Saffron Vinaigrette

Makes about 1 cup

The sea-saltiness of anchovies is a perfect foil for the tang of citrus in this lively dressing. Use it to dress radicchio, arugula, or other hearty greens.

2 tablespoons fresh lemon juice

1 teaspoon minced lemon membrane
   and pulp (see page 45)

1 tablespoon seasoned rice vinegar

2 teaspoons Dijon mustard

2 teaspoons anchovy paste

1 large garlic clove, pressed

1 thread saffron

⅓ cup olive oil

Combine all the ingredients in a small, deep bowl. Whisk until thoroughly mixed. Store in an airtight container in the refrigerator.

Red Chard Vinaigrette

Makes ½ cup

This crimson dressing has the nutritive authority of a leafy green vegetable and is delicious over pasta salad.

½ cup water

¼ cup white wine vinegar

1 bunch red Swiss chard

2 tablespoons fresh lemon juice

½ teaspoon sugar

1 tablespoon olive oil

Sea salt to taste

Pinch of minced fresh dill

Pink peppercorns for garnish (optional)

In a medium saucepan, bring the water and vinegar to a boil. Add the chard, cover, and cook over high heat for 5 minutes, or until the leaves are limp. Using a slotted spoon, transfer the chard to a sieve. Hold the sieve over the pan and press the chard with the back of a large spoon to release the liquid. You should have ½ cup liquid. (Reserve the chard for another use; each leaf can be rolled into a small ball and coated with toasted sesame seeds for an appetizer.) Add the lemon, sugar, olive oil, salt, dill, and peppercorns, if desired, to the chard liquid. Mix well, cover, and refrigerate.

Ginger-Citrus Dressing

Makes 1 cup

Ginger and citrus together make a lively fresh dressing. When dashed on scallops, the taste is purely Thai! This is also an ideal topping for buckwheat noodles or rice.

2½ tablespoons grated fresh ginger

¼ cup low-salt soy sauce

2 tablespoons mirin (sweet sake) or dry sherry

1 teaspoon minced garlic

1 teaspoon Asian sesame oil

½ teaspoon red pepper flakes or chili oil

2 scallions, finely chopped

¼ teaspoon grated lemon zest

2 tablespoons fresh lemon juice

¼ cup fresh orange juice

¼ tablespoon minced orange and lemon membrane and pulp (see page 45)

Combine all the ingredients except the citrus membrane and pulp in a small saucepan and bring to a boil. Reduce heat and simmer for 2 minutes. Set aside to cool. Add the minced membrane and pulp just before serving.

HOT AND SOUR AIOLI

Makes 1½ cups

Sorrel's lemony tart taste is the "sour" part of this recipe, while horseradish is the hot part. This will brighten up cold poached fish.

½ cup sorrel leaves

½ cup water or low-salt vegetable broth

5 to 6 garlic cloves

1 egg

1 teaspoon fresh lemon juice

1 teaspoon Dijon mustard

¼ teaspoon grated fresh horseradish,
  or ½ teaspoon prepared horseradish

½ teaspoon salt

¼ teaspoon white pepper

6 tablespoons safflower oil

2 tablespoons almond oil

ut out and discard the central stalks of the sorrel and coarsely chop the leaves. In a small saucepan, bring the water or broth to a boil. Reduce heat to a simmer, add the sorrel, and cook for 5 minutes, or until limp. Let cool slightly, then place the sorrel leaves in a blender or food processor and puree, adding 1 teaspoon of water if needed. Pour into a bowl and set aside.

In the blender or food processor, chop the garlic. Add the egg, lemon juice, mustard, horseradish, salt, and pepper. Blend until smooth. With the machine running, slowly drizzle the oils into the mixture in a fine stream until the mixture reaches the consistency of mayonnaise. Let cool, then stir in the sorrel puree and combine thoroughly. Store in an airtight container in the refrigerator until ready to use.

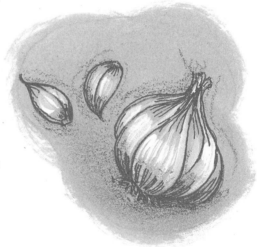

ARUGULA-WATERCRESS PESTO

Makes 1 cup

Peppery watercress makes a tasty topping for little pizzas or steamed winter vegetables.

¼ cup packed arugula leaves

¼ cup packed watercress leaves, stems trimmed

3 garlic cloves

¼ cup olive oil, plus 3 tablespoons olive oil

¼ cup fresh lemon juice

¼ teaspoon salt

¼ cup grated Parmesan cheese

2 tablespoons pine nuts

Salt and freshly ground pepper to taste

Place all the ingredients except the 3 tablespoons oil, salt, and pepper in a blender or food processor and process to a coarse puree. Season with salt and pepper. Pour into an airtight container. Add the remaining 3 tablespoons oil to cover the pesto with a thin layer. Cover and refrigerate. Spoon off the top layer of oil just before using.

HOT PEANUT SAUCE

Makes ½ cup

When peanut butter is combined with coconut milk and fresh lime juice, the effect is tropical and exotic. Serve on hot or cold soba or whole-wheat noodles.

¼ cup chunky natural peanut butter

¼ cup low-fat coconut milk

3 tablespoons fresh lime juice

2 tablespoons minced fresh cilantro

1 tablespoon low-salt soy sauce

2 tablespoons packed brown sugar

Place all the ingredients in a blender or food processor and puree until smooth. Transfer to a small saucepan and heat until warm.

THREE-MUSTARD SAUCE
WITH MARIGOLD

Makes about ¾ cup

Use this dark golden sauce to garnish grilled meats, airy mashed potatoes, or cooked, strongly flavored leafy vegetables such as chard or kale.

1 cup nonfat chicken broth

1½ cups low-salt vegetable broth

½ cup dry white wine

2 tablespoons tequila

½ fennel bulb, trimmed and diced

2 teaspoons Dijon mustard

1 teaspoon whole-grain mustard

1 teaspoon Creole or spicy brown mustard

⅓ cup marigold or nasturtium petals, chopped

Freshly ground pepper to taste

Combine the broths, wine, and tequila in a heavy, medium saucepan. Boil over high heat for 10 minutes, then add the fennel and mustards. Continue to boil until reduced to ¾ cup, about 15 minutes. Lower heat and simmer until slightly thickened, about 3 minutes. Let cool and transfer to a blender or food processor. Add the flower petals and puree. Add the pepper.

Corn, Yam, and
ROASTED RED PEPPER PUREE

Makes about 1½ cups

A medley of Southwestern flavors makes a lovely puree to serve
with hot cornbread or corn cakes, or as a dip with pita wedges.

> 1 yam
>
> 2 red bell peppers, roasted, peeled,
> and chopped (see page 59)
>
> 1 cup fresh corn kernels, steamed
>
> 1 teaspoon minced fresh cilantro
>
> 1 vine-ripened tomato, chopped
>
> 2 teaspoons fresh lemon juice
>
> ½ teaspoon cumin seeds, crushed
>
> Salt and freshly ground pepper to taste

Quarter the yam. Place in a steamer over boiling water, cover, and cook for
5 minutes. Peel. Place the yam and all the remaining ingredients in a blender
or food processor and puree until smooth.

ORANGE AND JUNIPER BERRY SAUCE

Makes about 1¼ cups

Fresh, tart, and sweet flavors mingle in a sauce for grilled duck or roasted chicken.

1 cup fresh orange juice with pulp

1½ tablespoons cornstarch

1 tablespoon butter

¼ cup sugar

1 tablespoon grated orange zest

¼ teaspoon red pepper flakes

3 juniper berries, crushed

In a small bowl, whisk the orange juice and cornstarch together until the cornstarch dissolves.

In a heavy small saucepan, melt the butter over medium-high heat. Whisk in the sugar, orange zest, orange juice mixture, and pepper flakes. Continue to whisk until the sauce boils and thickens slightly, about 4 minutes. Add the berries at the last minute. Let cool.

Tangy Tofu Sauce

Makes 1 cup

When teamed with lime, garlic, and dill, tofu takes on a tangy taste. Use as a dip for artichokes or a sauce for broccoli or asparagus.

8 ounces soft tofu, rinsed and drained

2 tablespoons fresh lime juice

2 tablespoons Dijon mustard

2 tablespoons walnut oil

2 tablespoons minced fresh dill

1 teaspoon salt

Place all the ingredients in a blender or food processor and puree until creamy. Cover and refrigerate for at least 30 minutes.

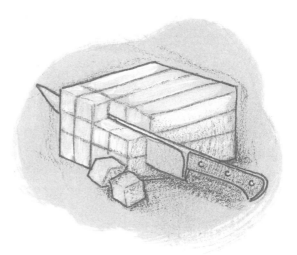

Sauces, Salsas, and Condiments

FRESH PAPAYA SAUCE

Makes 2 cups

Serve this sweet sauce with dessert crepes or spooned over sliced strawberries.

1 papaya, peeled and seeded

2 tablespoons sugar

1 teaspoon fresh lemon juice

1 teaspoon ground cinnamon

Dash of grated nutmeg

Dash of ground cardamom

Dice half the papaya and set aside. Place the remaining half in a blender or food processor and puree with the sugar, lemon juice, cinnamon, nutmeg, and cardamom until smooth. Stir in the diced papaya, cover, and refrigerate for at least 2 hours.

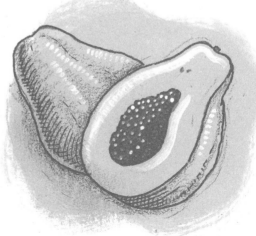

The Hot Flash Cookbook

RED ONION AND FINOCCHIO SALSA

Makes 4 cups

Finocchio, or sweet fennel, added to a Southwestern salsa makes a delicious topping for cold poached fish or cooked vegetables, or a filling for hot flour tortillas.

2 red onions, finely chopped

1 fennel stalk, finely chopped

½ cup minced fresh cilantro

3 ripe tomatoes, finely chopped

½ teaspoon salt

¼ teaspoon sugar

1 teaspoon fresh lime juice

1 cup minced fresh parsley

Freshly ground pepper to taste

Combine all the ingredients in a bowl and mix thoroughly. For a finer texture, pulse in a blender or food processor for a few seconds. Store in an airtight container in the refrigerator.

Fresh Fennel Coulis

Makes 1 cup

Licorice-laced and rich in garlic, this coulis is tarty with fish or crisp steamed vegetables.

> 3 tablespoons olive oil
>
> 2 fennel bulbs, trimmed and cut into julienne
>
> 1 garlic clove, crushed
>
> ½ teaspoon pepper
>
> 3 tablespoons white wine vinegar
>
> 1 teaspoon fresh lemon juice
>
> 1 tablespoon anisette liqueur

In a small, heavy saucepan over very low heat, heat the oil. Add the fennel, garlic, and pepper. Cover and cook, stirring occasionally, for 45 minutes. Add the vinegar, lemon juice, and anisette, and stir. Cook an additional 5 minutes. Set aside to let flavors develop. Reheat before serving, or serve cold.

FIERY ICED CAPSICUM SAUCE

Makes 2 cups

A cold sauce of yogurt is delicious with steamed fish or over rice
or coucous. Serve with fresh vegetable appetizers or as a substitute
for Mexican cream sauce on burritos or tacos.

1½ cups plain low-fat yogurt

2 ancho chiles

6 red bell peppers, roasted, peeled, and chopped
 (see page 59)

1½ teaspoons fresh lemon juice

⅛ teaspoon ground cumin

1 teaspoon kosher salt or to taste

Freshly ground pepper to taste

Put the yogurt in a sieve lined with a double thickness of cheesecloth and set
over a bowl. Refrigerate and let drain for several hours, or until slightly firm.
In a small saucepan, simmer the chiles in water to cover for about 5 minutes, or until tender. Drain, stem, and seed.

Place the yogurt, chiles, roasted peppers, lemon juice, cumin, salt, and pepper in a blender or food processor and puree until smooth.

Taste and adjust the seasoning. Cover and refrigerate for at least 2 hours.

DANDELIME SAUCE

Makes 1 cup

This vibrant sauce, rich in vitamin E, is a tasty topping for crisp steamed vegetables, shrimp, or white beans. Or, serve it as a dip with pita wedges.

> 1 egg yolk
>
> ½ cup minced dandelion leaves
>
> ¼ cup chopped whole scallions
>
> ¼ cup fresh lime juice
>
> 1 tablespoon Dijon mustard
>
> ½ teaspoon salt
>
> Freshly ground pepper to taste
>
> ¾ cup sesame or canola oil
>
> 2 teaspoons grated lime zest

In a blender or food processor, puree the egg yolk, dandelions, scallions, lime juice, mustard, salt, and pepper until smooth. With the machine running, gradually add the oil and process until the sauce is thick. Transfer to a bowl and stir in the lime zest. Store in an airtight container in the refrigerator for up to 5 days.

GINGER-ALMOND SAUCE

Makes 2 cups

This hearty paste of orange, ginger, and almond has a dash of fiery ginger that is perfect for lamb or pork. Serve over rice, pilaf, or cold poached fish.

1 cup almonds, toasted (see pages 52–53)

½ cup boiling water

½ cup fresh orange juice

1 tablespoon low-salt soy sauce

1 tablespoon minced orange membrane
   and pulp (see page 45)

1 teaspoon minced fresh ginger

½ teaspoon grated orange zest

Salt to taste

Grind the almonds in a blender or food processor, gradually adding the boiling water to make a paste. Transfer to a medium bowl. Add the remaining ingredients and mix well. Store in refrigerator up to 1 week.

Power Gomashio

Makes 1 cup

Goma is Japanese for sesame seed, and *gomashio* is a delightful mixture of seeds and sea salt, here embellished with a touch of herbs and licorice. Serve sprinkled over cold noodles or hot fish, or in soups.

¾ cup white sesame seeds

1 tablespoon salt

¼ teaspoon mustard seed

½ teaspoon dried basil

½ teaspoon dried garlic

½ teaspoon fenugreek seed

Heat a heavy skillet over medium heat. Add the sesame, mustard, and fenugreek seeds and toast, stirring constantly, for 2 minutes. Continue to cook, stirring constantly, until the seeds stop popping. Place in a mortar, nut grater, or blender and grind just until the seeds are partially ground and the oils have dampened the salt. Do not puree into a paste. Add the salt, basil, and garlic.

Sassy Pepper Pick-Me-Up

Makes ½ cup

This peppery mixture of vinegar, lime, and cayenne adds sparkle to stir-fry dishes, meats, or seafood.

> ½ cup distilled white vinegar
>
> 1 teaspoon salt
>
> 1 teaspoon sugar
>
> 1 teaspoon fresh lime juice
>
> 2 dried cayenne or serrano chiles, or 1 teaspoon cayenne pepper

In a small bowl, combine the vinegar, salt, sugar, and lime juice. Crush the chiles and soak in the vinegar mixture for 3 days, or until spicy. Cover and refrigerate.

Harissa the Firefighter

Makes ½ cup

Serve this thick, spicy paste with couscous, rice, bulgur, or other grains.

¼ **cup cayenne pepper**

2 **tablespoon ground cumin**

6 **garlic cloves**

1 **teaspoon salt**

½ **cup olive oil**

Using a mortar and pestle, crush the cayenne, cumin, garlic, and salt into a thick paste. In a small skillet over medium-high heat, heat the oil and add the paste; sauté for 5 minutes. Serve immediately, or cover and refrigerate.

Mint and Rose Hip Syrup

Makes 1¼ cups

This rosy-colored syrup is high in vitamin C. Pour it over sliced cantaloupe or papaya for an elegant dessert.

> **1 cup sugar**
>
> **2 cups water**
>
> **2 cups fresh rose hips, finely chopped**
>
> **2 fresh mint sprigs**

In a medium saucepan, combine the sugar and water. Bring to a boil and cook for 1 minute. Add the rose hips and mint. Lower heat and simmer gently for 1 hour, partially covered, adding more boiling water if needed. Strain through a sieve, pressing the pulp with the back of a spoon. Let cool.

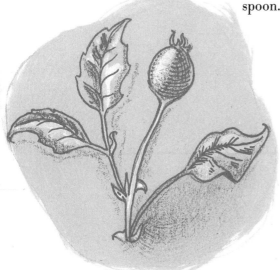

Sauces, Salsas, and Condiments

GINGER SYRUP

Makes ½ pint

This golden syrup enhances fresh fruit, pudding, custard, or rice.

½ cup chopped peeled ginger

1¼ cups boiling water

½ cup sugar

¼ cup candied ginger

Place the chopped ginger in a medium heatproof bowl. Add the boiling water and let sit for 30 minutes. Strain the infusion, then transfer to a saucepan and heat until warm. Add the sugar. When the sugar has dissolved, bring to a boil, then simmer gently over low heat until thick and syrupy. Let cool slightly and add the candied ginger. Pour into a glass jar, cover, and seal. Refrigerate.

Rose Hip Jelly

Makes 2 half pints

Garner rose hips from unsprayed rose bushes to make this beautiful, fragrant jelly rich with vitamin C.

2 pounds fresh rose hips, chopped

5 cups water

2 cups sugar or more as needed

3 tablespoons fresh lemon juice

Combine the rose hips and water in a large saucepan and boil for 1 hour, or until soft. Spoon into a jelly bag or a colander lined with a double thickness of cheesecloth and let drain into a bowl overnight. Measure the juice and add 2 cups of sugar for every 2½ cups juice. (Makes about 3 cups of juice.) In a heavy saucepan, bring to a boil, stirring to dissolve the sugar. Cover and boil until slightly thickened, about 2 minutes.

Skim off the surface scum and add the lemon juice. Pour the jelly into 2 hot sterilized half-pint jars, filling them to within ¼ inch of the top. Wipe the top with a clean cloth, then place a hot sterilized metal lid on top. Screw a metal band down tightly over the lid. Let cool and refrigerate.

BLACKBERRY-CRANBERRY RELISH

Makes 2 cups

This wonderful variation on cranberry sauce adds color and zest to turkey, chicken, or duck.

2 cups fresh blackberries	One 3-inch piece cinnamon stick
2 tablespoons balsamic vinegar	Pinch of salt
1 navel orange	15 whole cloves
¾ cup sugar	6 allspice berries
1½ cups water	1½ cups fresh cranberries

Place the blackberries in a shallow dish and sprinkle with the vinegar. Pare the zest from the orange with a sharp knife, cut it into 1-by-⅛-inch slivers, and set aside. Cut all the white outer membrane from the orange using a large, sharp knife. Mince the membrane and set aside. Cut the orange into segments, allowing each section to fall into the dish.

Combine the sugar, water, cinnamon stick, membrane, and salt in a heavy nonaluminum saucepan. Tie the cloves and allspice berries in a piece of cheesecloth or place them in a tea strainer; add the spices to the pan. Bring to a rolling boil and add the orange zest. Reduce heat to low and simmer for 10 minutes. Add the cranberries and orange segments and simmer for 1 more minute. Let cool for 5 minutes.

Pour the cranberry mixture over the blackberry mixture and mix gently. Let cool, then cover and refrigerate for at least 3 hours. Before serving, remove the spices and cinnamon stick.

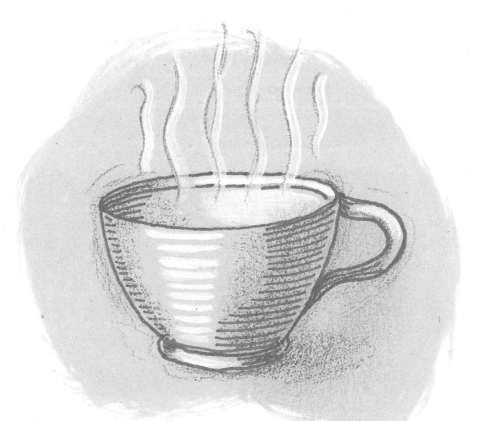

DRINKS

Nourish-Mint Tea

Makes 4 cups

This silky-smooth brew of mellow licorice, rose hips, and mint refreshes and invigorates.

> 1 teaspoon shredded licorice root
>
> 3 fresh mint leaves
>
> 1 tablespoon sugar
>
> 2 fresh rose hips, crushed
>
> 4 cups boiling water
>
> 1 whole clove

Put all the ingredients except the water and clove in a teapot. Add the water and let steep for 7 minutes. Add the clove and let steep 3 minutes longer. Strain and drink hot or cool.

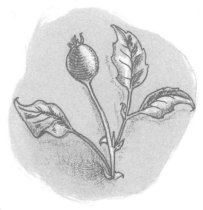

The Hot Flash Cookbook

Women's Tonic Tea

Makes 1 cup

The strong hormonal-regulating properties of this tea have a "euphoric" effect and boost both mental acuity and enthusiasm.

 1 tablespoon dried red raspberry leaf

 1 tablespoon dried nettle leaf

 1 tablespoon dried motherwort

 ½ tablespoon fennel seed

 1 cup boiling water

 1 whole clove

Add all the ingredients except the water and clove to a teapot. Add the water and let steep for 7 minutes. Add the clove and let steep for 3 minutes. Strain and serve.

Snap-To Tea

Makes 2 cups

Boiling water poured over dried herbs creates a delicious estrogen-rich brew that, unlike many teas, grows more flavorful the longer it steeps.

> 2 teaspoons fenugreek seed
>
> 1 teaspoon each sarsaparilla, dried camomile, dried comfrey leaf, dried motherwort, dandelion root
>
> ½ teaspoon ground licorice root
>
> ¼ teaspoon ground ginger
>
> ¼ teaspoon blue cohosh
>
> 2 cups boiling water

Put all the ingredients except the water in a teapot. Add the water and let steep for 20 minutes. Strain. Drink hot or cold.

Hot Flash Tea Blend

Makes 8 teaspoons

Herbal teas are free of harsh tannins. This deft blend of herbs has a lovely aroma as well as strengthening properties.

2 teaspoons dried or ground sage

2 teaspoons dried blessed thistle

1 teaspoon dried blue vervain

½ teaspoon dried rosemary

2 teaspoons dried motherwort

¼ teaspoon powdered ginseng

¼ teaspoon aniseed

Mix all the ingredients together. Store in an airtight container.

Brewed Hot Flash Tea: Add 1 cup boiling water to 1 teaspoon of the above blend. Cover and let steep for 30 minutes. Strain and drink no more than ¼ cup an hour as long as is needed.

Cool Vegetable Water

Makes 2 cups

Light, refreshing, and sugarless, this vegetable water, laced with lemon, is a healthy drink alternative.

2 cups water

2 cups leafy greens such as Swiss chard, kale, and spinach, chopped

Dash of ground cumin

2 squeezes of lemon juice

2 lemon slices

In a medium saucepan, bring the water to a boil. Add the greens and cook for 10 minutes. Strain, let cool, and refrigerate the liquid for 1 or 2 hours. Reserve the greens to use as an appetizer (see pages 67, 73, 87). Serve the liquid over ice with a dash of powdered cumin, a squeeze of lemon, and a lemon slice.

Ginger-Lime Tonic

Without the dong quai, this is a zesty, refreshing drink; with it, it is a natural means of balancing hormone levels and reducing hot flashes.

6 cups water

3 large limes

⅓ cup grated fresh ginger

½ piece dried dong quai,
  broken into pieces (optional)

½ cup sugar or honey

Bring the water to boil in a large nonaluminum saucepan. Remove from heat. Juice the limes, reserving the rinds, and set the juice aside. Add the rinds and ginger to the water and let stand for up to 1 hour. Add the dong quai, if using, and let steep for 1 to 2 minutes.

Add the lime juice and stir in the sugar or honey until dissolved. Strain into a pitcher and refrigerate until cold. Serve over ice.

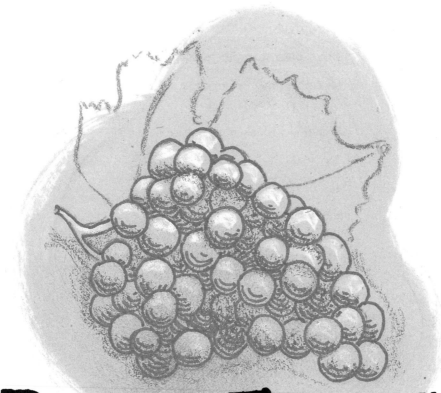

DESSERTS

BLACKBERRIES IN RED WINE SYRUP

Serves 2

The tangy sweet flavor and deep color of blackberries blend beautifully with the peppery wine flavor of the dark red syrup.

2 cups dry red wine

⅔ cup sugar

2 tablespoons orange zest strips

½ teaspoon minced orange membrane
  and pulp (see page 45)

¼ teaspoon black peppercorns

1 bay leaf

Dash of freshly grated nutmeg

1 tablespoon fresh lemon juice

2 cups fresh blackberries

In a 2-quart saucepan, bring the wine, sugar, zest, membrane and pulp, peppercorns, and bay leaf to a boil. Cook until reduced to 1½ cups, about 5 to 7 minutes. Strain the syrup into a bowl and discard the seasonings. Add the nutmeg and lemon juice and blend thoroughly.

Divide the berries between 2 bowls. Pour half of the syrup over each bowl of berries.

Pureed Mango with Mint

Makes 4 servings

Lush and tropical, this delicious, cold dessert is vivid in color and rich in vitamin E.

10 very ripe mangoes

⅛ teaspoon ground cardamom

¼ cup Cointreau or other orange liqueur

4 fresh mint sprigs for garnish

With a very sharp knife, carefully peel the mangoes and cut them away from the pit into chunks. Place in a blender or food processor and add the cardamom and liqueur. Puree briefly. Pour into individual serving glasses. Refrigerate for an hour, or until set. Garnish with sprigs of mint.

Mangoes in Tequila Tonic

Makes 4 servings

Delicious, slightly impudent, and replete with vitamin E, this
unusual dessert combines mangoes, tequila, and orange juice.

**4 plump mangoes (about 2 pounds),
     peeled and sliced from the pit**

¼ cup fresh orange juice

¼ cup distilled white vinegar

1 tablespoon olive oil

2 tablespoons tequila

2 teaspoons sugar

Salt and freshly ground pepper to taste

Garnish

Lettuce leaves

Unsprayed nasturtium blossoms

Arrange the mango slices on dessert plates. Mix the orange juice, vinegar,
olive oil, tequila, sugar, salt, and pepper in a small jar with a lid. Shake vigorously, then drizzle over the mangoes. Garnish with lettuce leaves and a flourish
of nasturtiums.

ALEXANDER DUMAS'S APRICOT COMPOTE

Makes 2 to 4 servings

Simplicity itself, this recipe has lived a long and glamorous life. Created by Dumas, author-cum-chef, the low-fat compote brims with flavor and nutrition, particularly vitamins A and E.

½ cup water

1 cup sugar

8 ounces fresh apricots, halved and pitted

Juice of 1 orange

In a heavy, medium saucepan, boil the water and sugar until thickened into a syrup, about 5 minutes. Add the apricots to the hot syrup and cook over medium heat for 3 minutes. Remove from heat and add the orange juice. Let cool before serving.

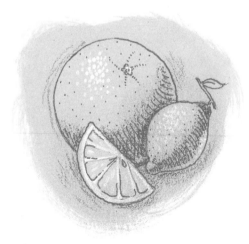

Desserts

Peach Paprika

Not too sweet, and definitely delicious, ripe peaches with lime is an unusual vitamin E-rich dessert.

2 firm, ripe peaches, peeled, pitted, and sliced

Juice of 1 lime

¼ teaspoon paprika

Fresh mint leaves for garnish

Arrange the peach slices on 2 serving plates and drizzle with the lime juice. Dust with paprika and garnish with mint leaves.

Glazed Clove Papaya

A sweet, cooling dessert rich in vitamin A: papayas glazed with a syrup of lime, honey, and cloves.

One 750-ml bottle late-harvest Gewürztraminer

20 whole cloves

¼ cup honey

⅛ teaspoon ground nutmeg

Dash of cayenne pepper

1 teaspoon balsamic vinegar

1 lime, peeled and thinly sliced

1 orange, peeled and thinly sliced

2 ripe papayas, peeled, halved, and seeded

Combine the wine, cloves, honey, nutmeg, cayenne, and vinegar in a nonaluminum saucepan and bring to a boil. Reduce to a simmer and add half of the lime and orange slices, reserving the other half for garnish. Cover and simmer over low heat until the liquid is thickened and reduced to about 1 cup. Strain and set aside.

Arrange 1 papaya half on each of 4 dessert plates. Fan the reserved citrus slices around each papaya half and drizzle with the glaze.

Glazed Brandied Grapefruit

Makes 4 servings

Grapefruit becomes dessert when it's sprinkled with brandy and flamed with brown sugar.

2 ruby red grapefruits

4 to 8 tablespoons packed dark brown sugar

4 teaspoons brandy

Preheat the broiler. Cut each grapefruit in half and remove any seeds. Carefully cut between the segments and skin with a grapefruit spoon or a paring knife. Drain off the accumulated juice.

Spread 1 to 2 tablespoons brown sugar over each grapefruit half and moisten with 1 teaspoon brandy. Place in a baking pan and broil for 5 to 7 minutes, or until the sugar is melted.

Candied-Ginger Applesauce

Makes 4 servings

The homespun appeal of apples, one of the top twenty-five vitamin E-bearing foods, is sparked by clove, ginger, and lemon. Serve as a dessert or a relish.

2 McIntosh apples, peeled and cored (reserve peels)

2 Granny Smith, Pippin, or other tart green apples, peeled and cored (reserve peels)

1 cup water

Juice of ½ lemon

½ cup packed brown sugar

½ teaspoon ground cinnamon

¼ teaspoon ground cloves

2 tablespoons minced candied ginger

¼ teaspoon grated fresh ginger

1 teaspoon butter (optional)

Cut the apples into wedges and combine with the water, lemon juice, sugar, cinnamon, and cloves in a medium, heavy pan. Cook over medium heat for 15 minutes, or until tender. Remove from heat and mash coarsely with a potato masher or puree in a blender. Add the candied and grated ginger and optional butter. Return to heat and cook for 3 minutes. Let cool slightly. Serve warm or cold.

Apple, Fig, and Blackberry Compote

Makes 6 to 8 servings

Apples and blackberries combine with plump and luxurious figs in this Indian summer dessert.

8 fresh figs, halved (about 1½ cups)

5 firm green or golden apples, peeled, cored, and cut into ¼-inch-thick wedges

2 cups blackberries

½ cup plus 3 tablespoons sugar

Finely grated zest of ½ lemon

1 tablespoon fresh lemon juice

½ cup water

½ cup crème fraîche or Gouda cheese

In a large bowl, combine the figs, apples, blackberries, sugar, lemon zest, juice, and water. Transfer the mixture to a medium saucepan and cook over low heat for 2 minutes. Cover and let cool to room temperature.

Serve with a dollop of crème fraîche or a slice of Gouda cheese.

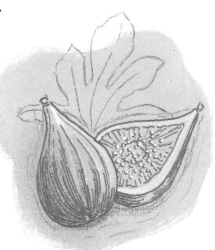

POACHED PEARS
IN BLOOD ORANGE SYRUP

Makes 4 to 6 servings

Firm Bartlett pears holds their shape during cooking. The juice of blood oranges provides a tart-sweet contrast to the subtle taste and texture of the pears.

2 cups dry red wine

1 cup water

1 cup fresh blood orange juice

¼ teaspoon fresh lemon juice

1 cup sugar

1 cinnamon stick

Dash of freshly grated nutmeg

½ vanilla bean, split lengthwise

4 to 6 Bartlett pears, peeled but stems left on

Combine the wine, water, orange juice, lemon juice, sugar, cinnamon, nutmeg, and vanilla in a large saucepan. Bring to a boil, then lower heat to a simmer. Slice the rounded bottom off each pear so it will stand upright. Add the pears, stems up, to the saucepan and poach for 15 minutes, or until tender. Using a slotted spoon, transfer the pears to serving dishes. Increase heat to high and cook to reduce the poaching liquid by half, about 15 minutes. Pour the sauce over the poached pears and serve.

Persian Bitterfruit

Makes 4 servings

The tang of grapefruit contrasts with cantaloupe's sweetness to create an invigorating mélange of fruit and spices, typically served as a Middle Eastern refreshment.

2 cantaloupes, halved and seeded

2 tablespoons Amaretto

2 ruby grapefruits, peeled and halved

**6 fresh mint leaves, finely julienned,
    plus 5 fresh mint sprigs for garnish**

1 teaspoon ground cardamom

Pinch of ground cumin

Scoop the melon flesh into balls. Set aside the shells to use as serving bowls. In a glass bowl, combine the melon balls and Amaretto. Squeeze the juice of one grapefruit half into the melon mix. Separate the remaining 1½ grapefruits into segments by hand. Do not trim away outer membrane. Add the grapefruit sections and julienned mint leaves to the melon ball mixture. Sprinkle the cardamom and cumin over the mixture and toss.

To serve, heap the fruit mix in the melon shells and garnish with mint sprigs.

CHILLED LICORICE-PEAR SOUP

Makes 6 to 8 servings

Used as a natural sweetening, licorice twigs add a cool, flavorful touch to this unusual dessert soup.

2¼ cups water

¼ teaspoon salt

4 tablespoons honey or packed brown sugar

2 licorice twigs (available in natural foods stores)

8 pears, peeled, cored, and diced

½ teaspoon minced fresh ginger

¼ teaspoon anise extract

Fresh mint sprigs for garnish

In a large stockpot, bring the water to a boil, then lower heat to a simmer. Add the salt, honey or brown sugar, and licorice; cook for 10 minutes to create a distinct licorice flavor.

Add the pears, ginger, and anise extract and continue to simmer for 4 minutes. Allow the mixture to cool. Transfer to a blender or food processor and puree until smooth. Garnish with mint sprigs and serve.

MangoPause Sorbet

Makes 3 cups

Look for fully ripe mangoes, plump to the touch, with a reddish blush to the skin. This refreshing tropical dessert is lovely in hot weather.

**Two 1-pound mangoes, peeled,
cut from the pit, and coarsely chopped**

½ cup sugar

6 tablespoons water

2 tablespoons fresh lime juice

**½ teaspoon minced lime pulp and membrane
(see page 45)**

In a blender or food processor, puree the mangoes. Pour the puree into a medium bowl.

Mix the sugar and water in heavy small saucepan. Stir over medium heat until the sugar is completely dissolved. Stir the syrup into the mango puree, then add the lime juice, pulp, and membrane and combine thoroughly.

Refrigerate the mango mixture for about 1 hour, or until completely chilled. Transfer to an ice cream maker and freeze according to the manufacturer's instructions.

Ruby Granita

There's only a hint of added sweetening in this refreshing Italian ice, which combines the juice of blood oranges with orange liqueur.

Juice of 12 blood oranges

2 tablespoons orange liqueur

2 tablespoons powdered sugar

½ teaspoon blood orange zest

1 tablespoon minced blood orange pulp (see page 45)

I n a large bowl, combine all the ingredients. Pour into a metal loaf pan and place in the freezer. Stir periodically until the mixture is frozen to a fine slush.

Cinnamon Licorice Granita

Makes 3 cups

Tired of hot tea? Try this icy blend of licorice and wine to bring a hot flash lull.

3 cups water

½ cup sugar

1 licorice twig

1¼ cups Merlot or Pinot Noir wine

½ teaspoon ground cinnamon

Combine the water and sugar in a large saucepan and heat to a simmer. Cover and cook for 5 minutes, stirring occasionally with the licorice twig. Do not allow the twig to steep, as the taste will become too strong. Stir in the wine and cinnamon. Let cool to room temperature. Pour into a metal loaf pan and place in the freezer for several hours, or until slushy, whisking it every hour to keep it smooth.

Blackberry-Coconut Sorbet

Makes 3 cups

This deep-colored sorbet is intensely rich in flavor and vitamin E.

⅓ cup water

6 tablespoons sugar

½ cup canned low-fat coconut milk,
  or ½ cup yogurt with 3 tablespoons
  dried coconut flakes

3½ to 4 cups fresh blackberries

2 tablespoons blackberry liqueur

In a medium saucepan, bring the water, sugar, and coconut milk to a boil. If using yogurt, eliminate the milk. Add 3 cups of the blackberries. Reduce heat and simmer for 3 to 4 minutes, or until the sugar is completely dissolved.

Pour the mixture through a fine-meshed strainer, pressing it with the back of a wooden spoon. Stir in the blackberry liqueur. If using yogurt, stir in. Refrigerate for 30 minutes. Freeze in an ice cream maker according to the manufacturer's instructions. Serve with the remaining ½ to 1 cup blackberries as garnish.

STICKY RICE
WITH STAR FRUIT

Makes 4 servings

Star fruit, or carambola, is mildly sweet and tangy. Here, a
festive array of star-shaped slices encircles sweet rice drizzled
with coconut sauce.

½ cups glutinous (sweet) rice

⅓ cups canned low-fat coconut milk, stirred

⅓ cup plus 3 tablespoons sugar

¼ teaspoon salt

3 star fruit, cut crosswise into ½-inch-thick slices

1 tablespoon sesame seeds, toasted
   (see page 55)

3 tablespoons sunflower seeds, toasted
   (see page 55)

Wash the rice thoroughly in cold water, changing the water several times until
it runs clear. Cover the rice in cold water and soak overnight. Drain the rice
well in a fine-meshed sieve. Add 2 inches of water to a stockpot and bring to a
simmer. Set the strainer over the simmering water, making sure it does not
touch the water. Cover with a dish towel and lid and steam for 30 to 40 minutes, or until tender. Check the water level from time to time, adding water as
needed.

While the rice is cooking, bring 1 cup of the coconut milk to boil in a small saucepan. Add the ⅓ cup sugar and the salt, stirring until sugar is dissolved. Set aside and keep warm.

Transfer the cooked rice to a large bowl and stir in the coconut milk mixture. Cover and let sit for at least 30 minutes, or up to 2 hours at room temperature. Meanwhile, slowly bring to a boil the remaining ⅓ cup coconut milk with the 3 tablespoons sugar, stirring occasionally. Cook for 1 minute. Transfer the sauce to a small bowl and refrigerate until cool and slightly thickened.

To serve, arrange star fruit slices in a circle on individual dessert plates. Spoon a small mound of rice in the center and drizzle with the sauce. Sprinkle with the sesame and sunflower seeds.

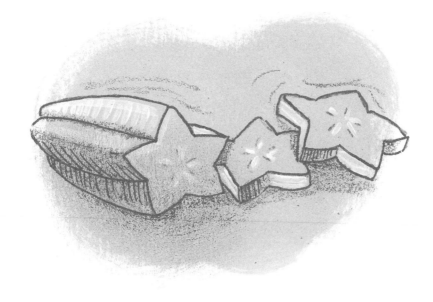

Picasso's Sugar Pane Apricot Puree
with Ricotta

Makes 4 to 6 servings

Adapted from a favorite dessert of Pablo Picasso, this treat is
visual as well as culinary. A jaunty "pane" of clear sugar acts as a
scoop for the rich ricotta.

1 pound nonfat ricotta cheese

1 cup sugar

1 cup water

APRICOT **1 cup dried apricots**

PUREE **2½ cups water**

¾ cup superfine sugar

3 tablespoons fresh lemon juice

Drain the ricotta overnight in a sieve lined with 2 layers of cheesecloth and placed over a bowl.

To make the sugar pane: Line a baking sheet with aluminum foil and butter it liberally. In a small, heavy pan, combine the sugar and water. Cook over high heat until bubbly and medium golden brown. Pour quickly onto the prepared baking sheet, tilting it to make the hot caramel form an "inkspill" shape. Let cool and break into irregular pieces that are as large as possible.

To make the apricot puree: Combine the apricots and 1½ cups of the water in a 2-quart saucepan and set aside for 2 hours. Add the remaining 1 cup water to the apricots and bring to a boil over medium heat. Cover, reduce heat to low, and cook for 20 minutes. Transfer to a blender or food processor and blend until smooth, stopping to scrape down the sides. Pour the puree into a large bowl. Stir in the sugar and the lemon juice. Let cool, then refrigerate for at least 1 hour.

To serve, mound a large spoonful of ricotta on each plate, spear a piece of sugar pane vertically into the mound, then drizzle all around with apricot puree.

Lavender Fool

Makes 4 servings

A colorful version of a traditional English dessert made with
gooseberries, this lavender-tinted berry-and-cream concoction by
Linda Hillel is a delicious way to replenish vitamin E.

1½ cups fresh blueberries

1½ cups fresh blackberries

⅓ cup sugar or to taste

3 tablespoons creme de cassis liqueur

1 cup Tapioca Cream (recipe follows)

Combine the berries and sugar in a large saucepan and cook over low heat,
stirring gently for about 10 minutes. Mash the berry mixture with the back of a
spoon and set aside to cool.

Gently fold the liqueur and fruit into the tapioca cream. Spoon into individual dessert dishes or into a large serving bowl. Refrigerate for 2 hours before
serving.

TAPIOCA CREAM

2 tablespoons instant tapioca

1 cup cold milk

2 egg whites

In a small saucepan, whisk together the tapioca and milk; let sit for 5 minutes. Place over medium-high heat and cook, stirring continuously for about 6 minutes, or until boiling and thick. Let cool completely.

In a large bowl, whip the egg whites until stiff peaks form. Fold into the cooled tapioca.

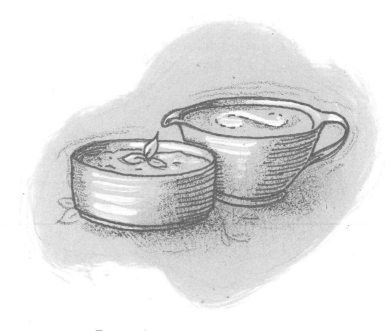

Desserts

Espresso-Yam Tarts

Makes two 6-inch tarts; serves 6

Yam puree, touched with espresso, cinnamon, and ginger, fills these tarts and supplies both vitamin E and calcium.

2 yams, peeled and quartered

½ cup maple syrup

1 teaspoon instant espresso powder

1½ cups nonfat milk

2 eggs, lightly beaten

2 tablespoons flour

1 teaspoon ground cinnamon

¼ teaspoon ground nutmeg

¼ teaspoon ground ginger

1/16 teaspoon ground cardamom

½ teaspoon salt

2 unbaked 6-inch tart shells

Fresh orange slices for garnish

Preheat the oven to 425°F. In a large, covered pot, steam the yams over boiling water until tender, about 10 minutes. Transfer to a blender or food processor and puree until smooth.

Pour the yam puree into a large bowl and add the syrup, espresso powder, milk, and eggs. Blend thoroughly. Stir in the flour, spices, and salt.

Pour the mixture into the tart shells and bake for about 20 minutes, or until a knife inserted in the center comes out clean. Let cool before serving.

Garnish with standing orange slices.

Lemon and Rose Hip Rice Pudding

Makes 2 to 4 servings

This soft, lemony custard brims with vitamin E, bioflavonoids, and vitamin C.

6 fresh rose hips, 2 crushed juniper berries, or ½ teaspoon minced lemon membrane and pulp (see page 45)

1⅔ cups water

1 cup long-grain white rice

¼ teaspoon salt

2 eggs, well beaten

⅓ cup packed brown sugar

¾ teaspoon grated lemon zest

2 tablespoons fresh lemon juice

¼ teaspoon vanilla extract

Ground cinnamon for sprinkling

If using the rose hips, cut them into slices. In a large, heavy saucepan, bring the water to a boil. Add the rice, rose hips, berries, or membrane and pulp, and salt. Bring back to a boil, then lower heat to a simmer. Cover and cook until the rice is tender, about 20 minutes. Remove from heat, beat in the eggs, and continue to beat for 1 or 2 minutes. Stir in the sugar, lemon zest, juice, and vanilla. Transfer to a serving dish. Sprinkle the top generously with cinnamon and let cool to room temperature. Serve now, or cover and refrigerate until cold.

Hazelnut Crescents

Makes 24 small crescents

Serve this cross between a scone and a cookie for dessert with fresh fruit or sorbet.

1½ cups (6 ounces) hazelnuts,
　　toasted and peeled (see pages 52–53)

4½ cups cake flour

½ cup cornmeal

1½ teaspoons baking powder

½ teaspoon baking soda

½ teaspoon salt

4 tablespoons cold unsalted butter, cut up

2 cups buttermilk

¼ cup packed brown sugar

1 teaspoon grated lemon zest

Preheat the oven to 350°F. Lightly butter a baking sheet. Grind the hazelnuts to a powder in a blender or food processor.

In a large bowl, combine the flour, cornmeal, ground hazelnuts, baking powder, baking soda, and salt. Mix well. With a pastry blender or 2 knives, cut in the butter until the mixture resembles coarse meal. Sprinkle the buttermilk over the surface of the dough a little at a time and stir into the flour. The dough should be soft.

On a lightly floured surface, pat the dough into a circle, then roll it out to a ½-inch thickness. Cut into pinwheels. With a metal spatula, transfer each arc to the baking sheet and pull slightly into a crescent shape. Sprinkle the scones with brown sugar and lemon zest. Bake for 10 to 15 minutes, or until firm and golden brown. Serve warm.

Note: For a shiny, chewier crust, brush the surface with 1 egg yolk mixed with 4 tablespoons milk before baking. If a softer crust is preferred, brush with milk after the crescents come out of the oven.

MIDLIFE TRIFLE

Makes 4 servings

A light but creamy coconut-flavored tapioca is layered with sponge cake, mango slices, and lime sauce.

TAPIOCA

1 egg white

6 tablespoons sugar

3 tablespoons instant tapioca

2 cups nonfat milk

1 egg yolk

1 teaspoon coconut extract

¼ teaspoon grated lime zest

¹⁄₁₆ teaspoon minced lime membrane and pulp (see page 45)

1 teaspoon fresh lime juice

LIME
SAUCE

½ cup sugar

½ cup water

Juice of 5 fresh limes

⅛ teaspoon minced lime pulp and membrane (see page 45)

MANGO CRUMBLE

One 9-inch sponge cake

2 mangoes

½ cup unsweetened shredded coconut, toasted

To make the topping: In a small bowl, beat the egg white until foamy, then add 3 tablespoons of the sugar and beat until stiff peaks form. Set aside.

Whisk the instant tapioca, the remaining 3 tablespoons sugar, the milk, and the egg yolk in a saucepan over medium heat for 5 minutes, or until the mixture reaches a full boil. Remove from heat. Quickly add the coconut extract, lime zest, membrane and pulp, juice, and egg white mixture and whisk until blended.

To make the sauce: In a small, heavy saucepan, boil the sugar and water until as thick as honey, about 3 minutes. Thin to the desired consistency by drizzling in the lime juice. Add the membrane and pulp. Let cool for 1 hour, or until thick and shiny.

Slice the sponge cake in half horizontally. Peel the mangoes and cut the flesh away from the pit in thin slices.

In a large glass bowl, place 1 layer of the cake and top with half of the mango slices, one third of the tapioca, and half of the sauce. Repeat. Top with the remaining tapioca and the toasted coconut. Cover and refrigerate for several hours before serving.

BLUEBERRY-APRICOT MERINGUE CLOUD

Makes 6 to 8 servings

A culinary treasure so showy that its light, low-fat nutritional advantage is easy to overlook.

MERINGUE	5 large egg whites (about ⅔ cup)
	½ teaspoon cream of tartar
	1 cup sugar
	1 teaspoon vanilla extract

FRUIT PUREE	Fresh apricots, halved and pitted (3 cups)
	¼ cup Cointreau or other liqueur
	¼ cup sugar
	3 cups fresh blueberries

To make the meringue: Preheat the oven to 300°F. Oil and lightly flour a baking sheet.

In a large bowl, combine the egg whites and cream of tartar. Beat until frothy. Gradually beat in the sugar, 1 tablespoon at a time, until all the sugar is incorporated and the whites form stiff peaks. Beat in the vanilla.

Swirl the meringue in an 8-inch-wide mound onto the prepared baking sheet, forming peaks on top.

Bake the meringue until it is firm and pale gold, about 1¼ hours. Let cool completely. Transfer to a plate, cover, and refrigerate for up to 24 hours.

To make the puree: In a blender or food processor, puree the apricots, orange liqueur, and sugar.

Coat the top of the meringue with half the apricot puree and scatter with half the blueberries.

Cut the meringue into 6 to 8 wedges. Place 1 wedge on each dessert plate and drizzle with some apricot sauce and sprinkle with some berries.

FLOURLESS LEMON CORDIAL CAKE

Makes 6 to 8 servings

This dense, chewy almond cake, sprinkled with Cointreau or Amaretto, is perfect for those who are allergic to wheat.

1½ cups (7 ounces) slivered almonds

½ cup plus 3 tablespoons powdered sugar, sifted

4 large eggs, separated

3 tablespoons Cointreau or Amaretto liqueur

5 teaspoons packed grated lemon zest

Juice of 3 lemons (about ¼ cup)

½ teaspoon ground cinnamon

Pinch of salt

Zest curls for garnish

Preheat the oven to 375°F. Butter and flour an 8-inch round cake pan and line the bottom with waxed paper.

In a blender or food processor, grind the almonds with 2 tablespoons of the sugar. Add the egg yolks, liqueur, 2 tablespoons of the sugar, lemon zest and juice, cinnamon, and salt to the almond mixture and blend until smooth.

In a large bowl, beat the egg whites until they form soft peaks. Gradually add 4 tablespoons of the sugar, beating until stiff but not dry.

Gently fold half of the egg whites into the almond mixture, then fold in the remaining half. Spread the batter in the prepared pan and bake for about 35 minutes, or until a cake tester comes out clean. Let cool completely in the pan on a wire rack. Turn out on a serving plate. Dust with the remaining 3 tablespoons powdered sugar and sprinkle with the zest curls.

BIBLIOGRAPHY

Brickoin, Mark, and the editors of *Prevention* magazine. *Nutrition Advisor*. New York: MJF Books, 1993.

Brown, J. K., "A Cross-Cultural Exploration of the End of the Childbearing Years"; J. Griffen, "Cultural Models for Coping with Menopause"; and A. L. Wright, "Variation in Navajo Menopause: Toward an Explanation." In *Changing Perspectives on Menopause*, edited by A. M. Voda, M. Dinnerstein, and S. R. O'Donnel. Austin, Tex.: University of Texas Press, 1982.

Consumer Reports 7, No. 12, Dec. 1995. "Phytochemicals: Drugstore in a Salad?"

Cutler, Winnifred B., and Garcia, Celso-Ramon, M.D. *Menopause: A Guide for Women and Those Who Love Them*. New York: W. W. Norton & Company, 1992.

Erichsen-Brown, Charlotte. *Medicinal and Other Uses of North American Plants*. New York: Dover Publications, 1979.

Espinoza, Edgard O., Dr.; Mann, Mary-Jacques, M.F.S.; and Bleasdell, Bob, Ph.D. "The Ranges of Arsenic and Mercury Concentrations in Herbal Balls" (chart). *The New England Journal of Medicine*, Sept. 21, 1995.

Gillteman, Ann Louise. *Super Nutrition for Menopause*. New York: Pocket Books, 1993.

Greenwood, Sadja, M.D. *Menopause Naturally: Preparing for the Second Half of Life*. Volcano, Calif.: Volcano Press, 1988.

Henkel, Gretchen. *Making the Estrogen Decision*. Los Angeles: Lowell House, 1992.

Ito, Dee. *Without Estrogen: Natural Remedies for Menopause and Beyond*. New York: Crown Paperbacks, 1994.

Jern, Helen Z., M.A., M.D. *Hormone Therapy of the Menopause and Aging*. Springfield, Ill.: Charles C. Thomas, 1973.

Lark, Susan M., M.D. *The Menopause Self Help Book*. Berkeley, Calif.: Celestial Arts, 1990.

Lee, John R., M.D. *Natural Progesterone: The Multiple Roles of a Remarkable Hormone.* Sebastapol, Calif.: BLL Publishing, 1993.

Lock, Margaret. *Encounters with Aging: Mythologies of Menopause in Japan and North America.* Berkeley, Calif.: University of California Press, 1993.

Miksicek, R. J. "Commonly Occurring Plant Flavonoids Have Estrogenic Activity." *Molecular Pharmacology* 44, July 1993: 37–43.

Multidisciplinary Perspectives on Menopause, vol. 592. Annals of the New York Academy of Sciences, 1990.

Nachtigall, Lila, M.D., and Heilman, Joan Rattner. *Estrogen: The Facts Can Change Your Life.* New York: Harper & Row, 1986.

Perry, Susan, and O'Hanlan, Katherine A., M.D. *Natural Menopause: The Complete Guide to a Woman's Most Misunderstood Passage.* Menlo Park, Calif.: Addison-Wesley Publishing, 1993.

Taylor, Dena, and Sumrall, Amber Coverdale, eds. *Women of the 14th Moon: Writings on Menopause.* Freedom, Calif.: The Crossing Press, 1994.

Ulene, Dr. Art, and Dr. Val. *The Vitamin Strategy.* Berkeley: Ulysses Press, 1994.

U. S. Congress Office of Technology Assessment. *The Menopause, Hormone Therapy and Women's Health.* OTA-BP-88. Washington, D.C.: U.S. Government Printing Office, 1992.

INDEX

The Hot Flash Cookbook

Index

269

The Hot Flash Cookbook

5575